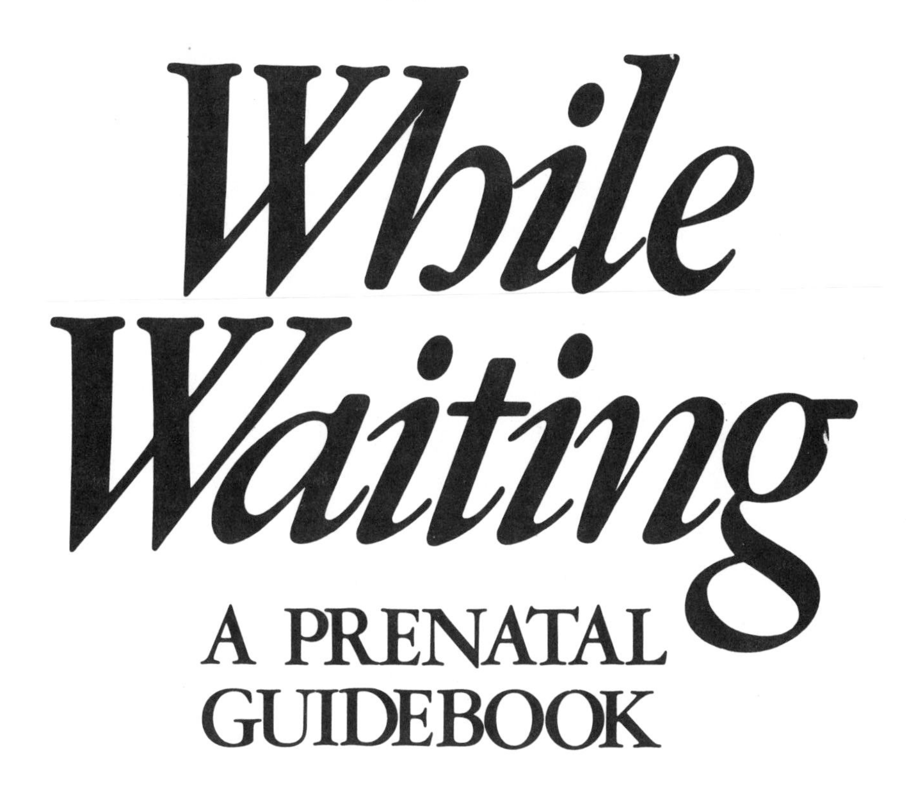

While Waiting

A PRENATAL GUIDEBOOK

George E. Verrilli, M.D., F.A.C.O.G.
Anne Marie Mueser, Ed.D.

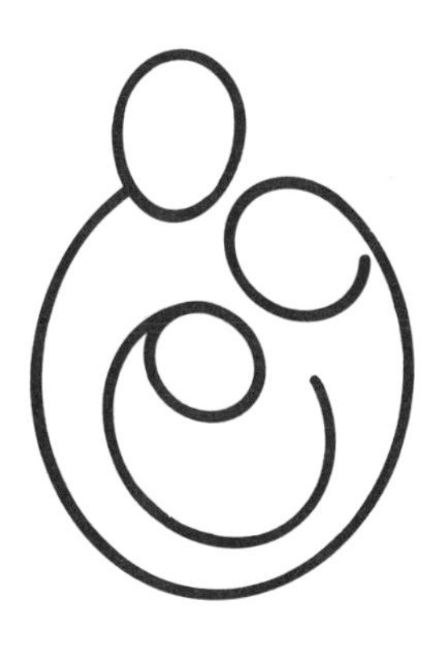

ST. MARTIN'S PRESS / NEW YORK

35 34 33 32 31 30 29 28 27 26 25 24

Library of Congress Cataloging in Publication Data

Verrilli, George E.

While waiting.

1. Pregnancy. 2. Childbirth. 3. Prenatal care.

I. Mueser, Anne Marie. II. Title.

RG525.V45 618.2'4 81-9008

ISBN 0-312-86773-5 AACR2

Manufactured in the United States of America

Editor: Barbara Anderson
Design and Production: Harry Chester Associates
Illustrations: George Wildman and Kristina Nörgaard
Consultants: Eileen Conde, RN, CCE; Chris Kilmer, RN, NAACOG; Janet McKee Marshall, CNM; Barbara M. Perkins, RN; Elaine P. Wood, RN, NAACOG; Cecilia L. Worth, RN, CCE

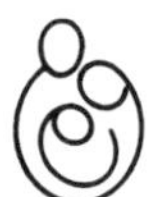

ACKNOWLEDGMENTS

During the various stages of development and delivery of WHILE WAITING, many people helped. The authors especially wish to thank:

—the administration and staff at Northern Dutchess Hospital, for providing a supportive atmosphere for family-centered childbirth and setting for our work

—the many doctors, nurses, midwives, and the more than 250,000 women and their partners who have used WHILE WAITING

—Andrea Greaney, whose waiting for her son Michael went almost by the book, for her page-by-page critique

—Bianca's mother, Chris, for her encouragement and support

—Richard P. Perkins, MD, FACOG, for his review of the manuscript and helpful suggestions

—Cecelia Worth, for her contribution to the content of WHILE WAITING, as well as for the title

—our editor, Barbara Anderson, whose support and encouragement never wavered

—Harry Chester and his staff, whose creative efforts and patience helped bring this book to being a reality at last.

TABLE OF CONTENTS

About the Authors

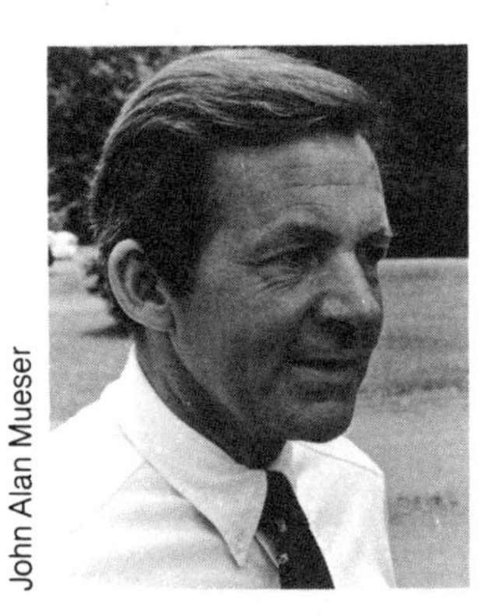
John Alan Mueser

George Verrilli, a practicing obstetrician for more than 20 years, has delivered more than 6,000 babies. He received his M.D. degree from the University of Turin, and is a Fellow of the American College of Obstetricians and Gynecologists.

Dr. Verrilli is Chief of Obstetrics and Gynecology at Northern Dutchess Hospital in Rhinebeck, New York, where he has been a member of the hospital's Board of Directors since 1968. Under Dr. Verrilli's leadership, the obstetrical service at Northern Dutchess pioneered in implementing family-centered childbirth practices in a hospital setting.

Dr. Verrilli has a daughter, Bianca, born December 31, 1982, and three grown sons.

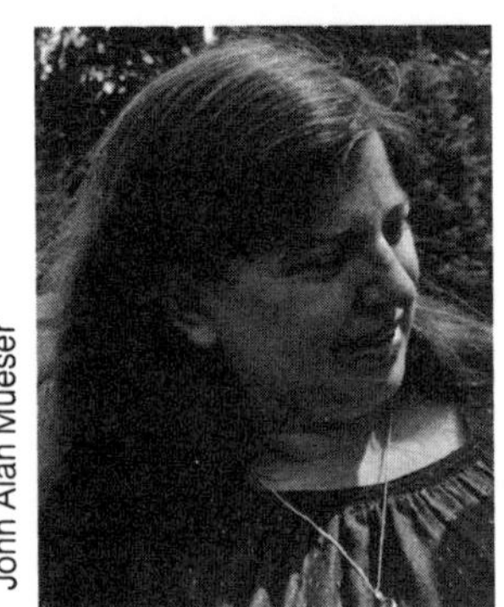
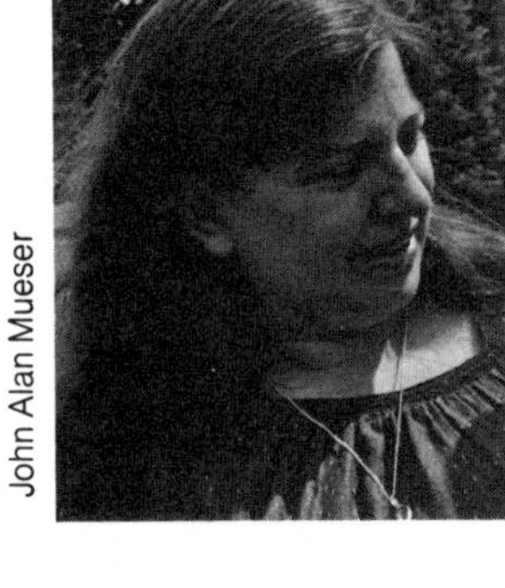
John Alan Mueser

Anne Marie Mueser, a writer and teacher for more than 15 years, has worked in elementary schools as a classroom teacher and reading specialist, and in clinical settings with learning disabled and dyslexic children. Formerly an Associate Professor of Education at Teachers College Columbia University, Dr. Mueser left the university in 1978 to devote her professional energies to her career as a writer. She is the author of numerous children's books and educational materials, and she occasionally works on a novel.

Her first child, Ánna Máire, was born in August of 1980. Dr. Mueser is Program Coordinator for Aer Lingus/Horses & Ireland equestrian holidays. She and her daughter divide their time between their home in Dutchess County, New York, and County Galway, Ireland.

On the Cover

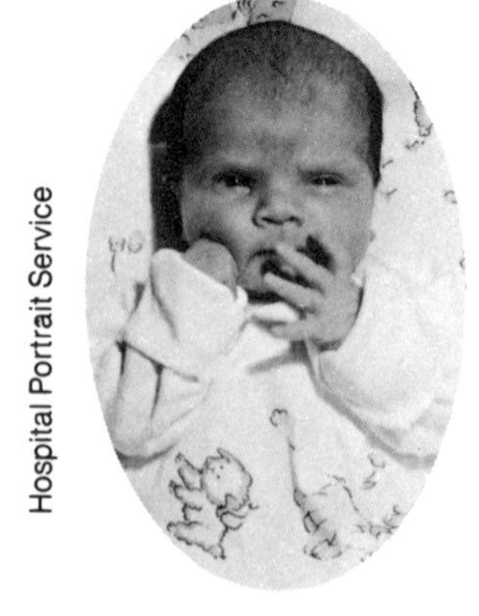
Hospital Portrait Service

Ánna Máire Mueser — delivered by Dr. Verrilli —arrived on August 13, 1980, at 3:07 p.m. She weighed 6 pounds 6 ounces and was 18 inches in length. The cover picture was taken a day later by a member of the Mothers' Club of Northern Dutchess Hospital, under contract with Hospital Portrait Service.

Note the shape of Ánna Máire's head, the slightly swollen eyelids, the wrinkled skin on her hands, and the way one hand is curled into a little fist. These are all typical characteristics of a newborn. The picture on the back cover of WHILE WAITING was taken when Ánna Máire was ten months of age.

INTRODUCTION

While Waiting: A Prenatal Guidebook contains many of the things I discuss with women who come to my office for obstetrical care. Annie Mueser, who listened to most of what I told her while she was pregnant, has drawn on her many years of experience as a writer and teacher to put this information in its present form.

This material is designed to be used for a reference. In the sections "Coping With Bodily Changes" and "For Your Information" the topics are arranged alphabetcially so you can easily locate what you need. You don't have to sit down and read the entire book from cover to cover, although we hope you'll want to do that, too.

We suggest that you use this book as if you were having a conversation with your doctor or nurse midwife. Bring it to your appointments, and if you have questions about anything you've read, be sure to ask. Your healthcare team, of course, knows you personally, and may modify some of the suggestions to fit your particular situation. And, remember that professionals do differ in their opinions regarding certain of these matters. Our guidelines are offered as suggestions, not absolutes. Use them to help you work with your prenatal care providers. The book contains pages to keep track of your appointments, diet, questions, and other important items as your pregnancy progresses. We hope you'll find this material useful WHILE WAITING.

George E. Verrilli, M.D.

Publisher's Note

The suggestions, procedures, and other materials in this book are not intended as a substitute for consultation with your physician. Medical supervision is recommended for prenatal care and any other matters concerning your health.

This book belongs to:

Doctor's Name:

Address:

Telephone:

Hospital:

Address:

Telephone:

Emergency Numbers:

Section One

WORKING WITH YOUR HEALTHCARE TEAM

The First Visit / Personal History / Physical Exam / Prenatal Laboratory Tests / When Is the Baby Due? / Followup Visits / Between Visits / Important Warning Signs / Appointment Record / Questions and Notes / How Your Baby Grows

If you are pregnant, you probably are already going to the professional of your choice for prenatal care. However, if you have not yet chosen a doctor or midwife, we suggest that you do so as soon as possible.

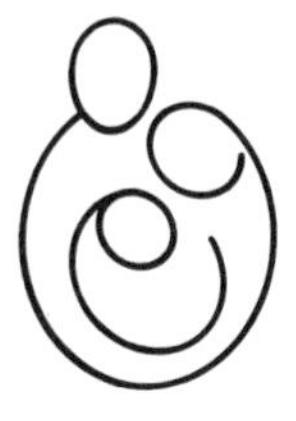

FIRST PRENATAL VISIT

Many prenatal care providers welcome both parents at visits to the office. You may, of course, come to your appointment by yourself. You may wish to bring another person close to you with a special interest in your pregnancy. Feel free to ask any questions you might have about this.

The first visit is designed to gain a picture of your general condition going into this pregnancy.

PERSONAL HISTORY

You will be asked to provide facts about your health and that of the baby's father. Hereditary possibilities (twins, for example, or a family history of certain diseases) are discussed. You will be asked about your previous pregnancies (including miscarriages), if any, and about your social and work background.

PHYSICAL EXAM

The examination includes a careful assessment of your breasts, throat, lungs, kidneys, liver, heart and blood pressure, bladder, and uterus in regard to your developing pregnancy. Your pelvic measurements are checked at this time.

PRENATAL LABORATORY TESTS

A number of laboratory tests are done to obtain information needed to monitor your health and that of your developing baby. These tests include:

- A urine test for the presence of protein, glucose, and nitrates, to keep track of kidney function.
- A Pap Smear (unless you have had one done within the past year) to screen for cervical cancer.
- A blood test to check for a number of different things:
  - — red blood cell level to see if you and your baby are getting enough oxygen (Hematocrit — HCT).
  - — your blood type and whether or not you carry the Rh factor.
  - — whether or not you carry antibodies to Rubella (German Measles).
  - — syphilis (this test is required by the State).
- Any other tests that might be specifically indicated for your particular circumstances, at your request or the suggestion of your medical team.

WHEN IS THE BABY DUE?

There is a formula for estimating this date, but keep in mind that it is only an estimate. It is perfectly normal for a baby to be born as much as two weeks before or after this date. Your body and your baby will decide the right time.

To estimate the due date, add seven days to the first day of your last menstrual period. Then count back three months.

An average pregnancy is 280 days, or 40 weeks from the first day of the last menstrual period if your cycle is regular. If figured from the time of ovulation, an average pregnancy is 266 days. You can add or subtract one day for each day that your menstrual cycle is longer or shorter than the average length of 28 days.

Another way to estimate your baby's due date is to add five months to the time you first feel your baby move.

FOLLOWUP VISITS

During these visits the doctor or nurse midwife will discuss with you the progress of your pregnancy and any problems that you might have.

The following items are checked and noted each visit:

Weight
Blood Pressure
Baby's Heart (FH)
Level of Your Growing Uterus (Height of the Fundus — HOF)
Urine (Please bring with you a sample of your first urine of the morning. The sample should be refrigerated if your appointment is later in the day. If you can't refrigerate it bring it anyway.)

During the ninth month, your office visits will include preparation for labor and delivery, and an internal examination to check the condition of your cervix (effacement and dilation), the baby's position relative to your pelvic opening (station), and the baby's presenting part.

If you have questions about any of these procedures or the findings, please ask.

BETWEEN VISITS

If you have any problems of a medical nature—for example, fever, chills, bladder or bowel difficulties, sore throat or cold, bleeding, dizziness, spots before your eyes, tingling or numbness—call your prenatal care provider.

If medication is required, you must take one that is safe during pregnancy. So, it's best to check with the professionals providing your prenatal care before taking any medication during your pregnancy—even something you've routinely taken in the past, or medication prescribed by another doctor.

To keep you and your baby healthy, it's important that you and your prenatal caregivers work together.

IMPORTANT

Any of the following signs may be a warning that you need medical help. Call the doctor right away if you experience any of these.

****severe headache**
****blurring of vision or spots before your eyes**
****severe stomach pain or cramps, perhaps with nausea or diarrhea**
****marked swelling in your upper body (face or hands)**
****a sudden weight gain in just a few days**
****vaginal bleeding**
****a gush or flow of watery fluid from your vagina**
****regular contractions, getting stronger as time progresses**
****marked decrease or stopping of fetal movement you feel (from the fifth month on)**

Do not hesitate to call, even if you fear you may be bothering someone about something that might turn out to be unimportant. Remember, it's better to be safe than sorry.

APPOINTMENT RECORD

Date	Time	Weight	Blood Pressure	Urine	HOF	Other

Questions and Notes

Questions and Notes

HOW YOUR BABY GROWS

The following section of WHILE WAITING contains a brief, month-by-month description of the characteristics of a developing baby. The information offered here is based on average development. Although no two pregnancies are exactly alike, it will give you some idea of the nature and sequence of changes going on within your body.

Each page provides a place for your own notes as your pregnancy progresses. Use this space, if you wish, to jot down things that matter to you personally. You can keep track of your pregnancy's important milestones — for example, the first time you feel your baby move, or when you first notice Braxton-Hicks contractions. If the perfect name for your baby comes to mind, write it down. Describe any experiences, thoughts, or feelings you want to be sure to remember later. These are your pages. Use them as you choose.

The First Two Weeks

Your baby's life and growth begin at the moment a sperm joins the ripe ovum (egg) in one of your fallopian tubes. These two cells fuse and become one. The cell formed by the united sperm and egg — although it is no larger than the dot at the end of this sentence — contains the potential for everything your baby will become.

Within about half an hour, the cell formed by the joined sperm and ovum divides into two cells. The cells continue to divide as they travel toward the uterus. By the end of the first week to ten days, the cluster of cells completes its journey down the fallopian tube and attaches to the uterine wall.

The cells continue to divide at a very rapid rate. Those which will become the placenta grow against the uterine wall. The placenta connects to the little developing form by the umbilical cord. The cord brings nourishment from your body to your baby, while carrying off wastes from the baby so that your body can dispose of them.

Third and Fourth Weeks

Even before you may know for sure that you are pregnant, your baby's central nervous system, heart, and lungs start to develop. The tiny heart begins to beat.

By the end of the fourth week, the baby is about 3/16 of an inch long. Although distinct facial features are not yet apparent, the face is beginning to form and dark circles mark where the eyes will be.

Second Month

As the second month begins, your baby's ears are starting to develop. Each ear begins as a little fold of skin at the side of the head. Tiny buds that eventually will grow into arms and legs are forming. By this time, the brain and the spinal cord are already well formed. The head is large in proportion to the rest of the body.

At the end of eight weeks, your baby is about an inch long and weighs about 1/30 of an ounce. Now the arms and legs are beginning to show distinct divisions, including fingers and toes. The little buds that will become fingers already have fingerprints.

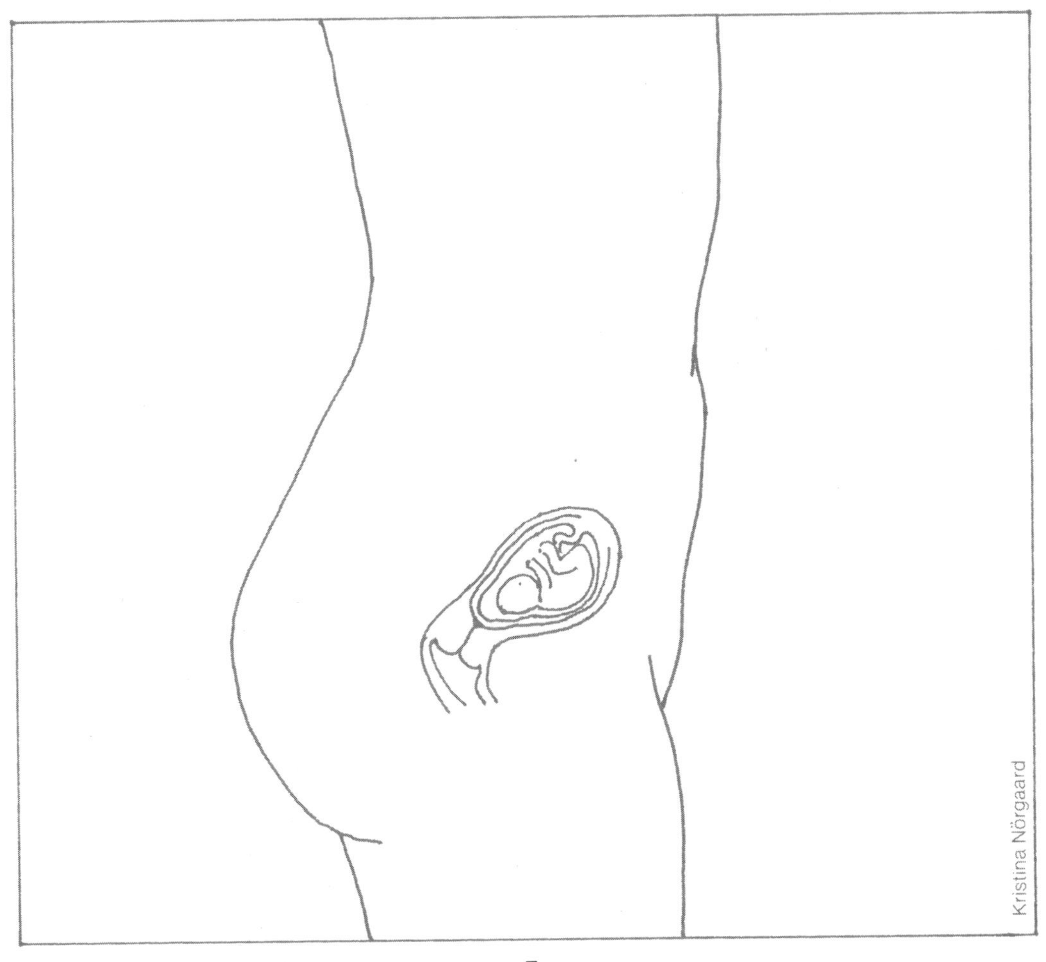

Third Month

By the end of three months, your baby is about three inches long and weighs about one ounce. The arms, with hands and fingers, and the feet, with toes, are fully formed. Fingernails and toenails are beginning to develop and the external ears are formed by this time. The beginnings of teeth are forming in the tiny jawbones.

The external sex organs are apparent by this time, and the internal sex organs are developing as well. If your baby is a boy, his testicles already contain sperm. If your baby is a girl, her ovaries already contain ova. So, even before this baby is born, the promise of the future generation is already present in these tiny cells.

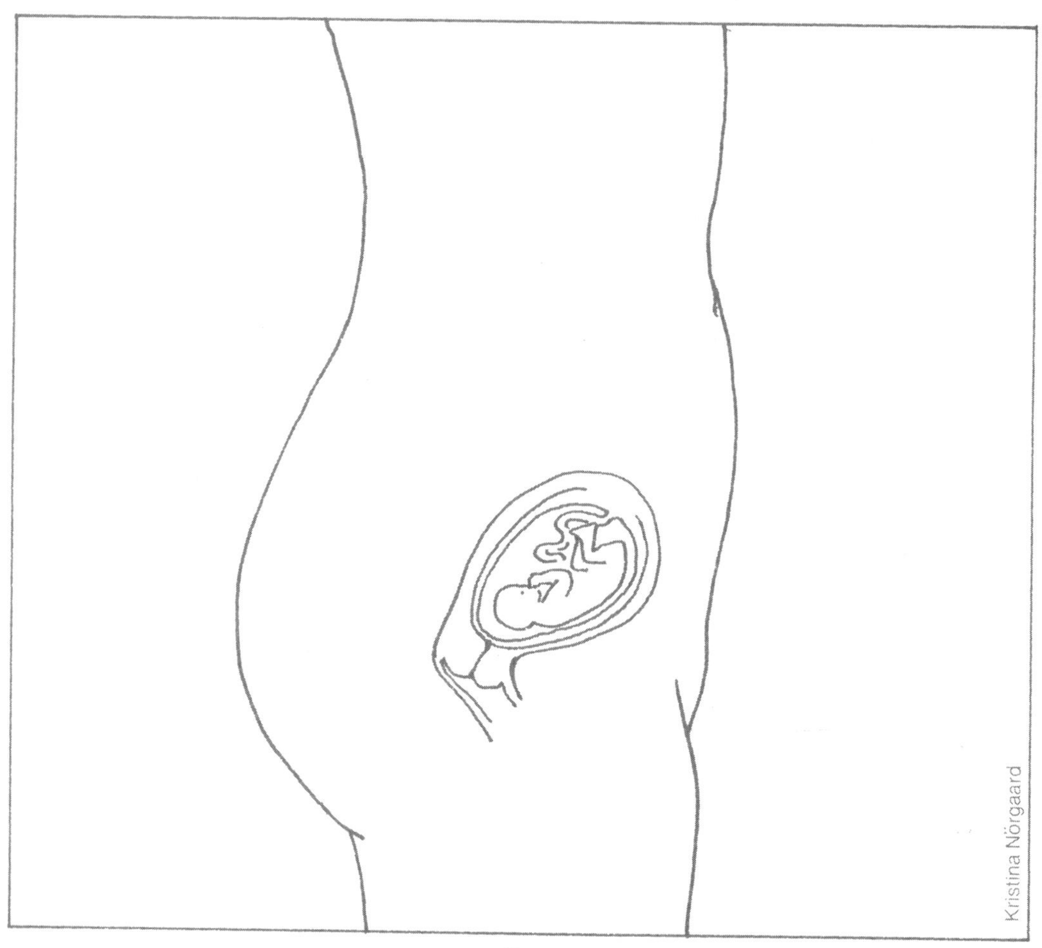

THE SECOND TRIMESTER

Fourth Month

Your baby's heartbeat can now be heard using a special stethoscope. Compared to the rest of the body, your baby's head seems very large at this point. Your baby's length will increase rapidly during this month.

By the end of the fourth month, your baby is about seven inches long and weighs about four ounces. The baby already has eyebrows and lashes and can suck his or her thumb.

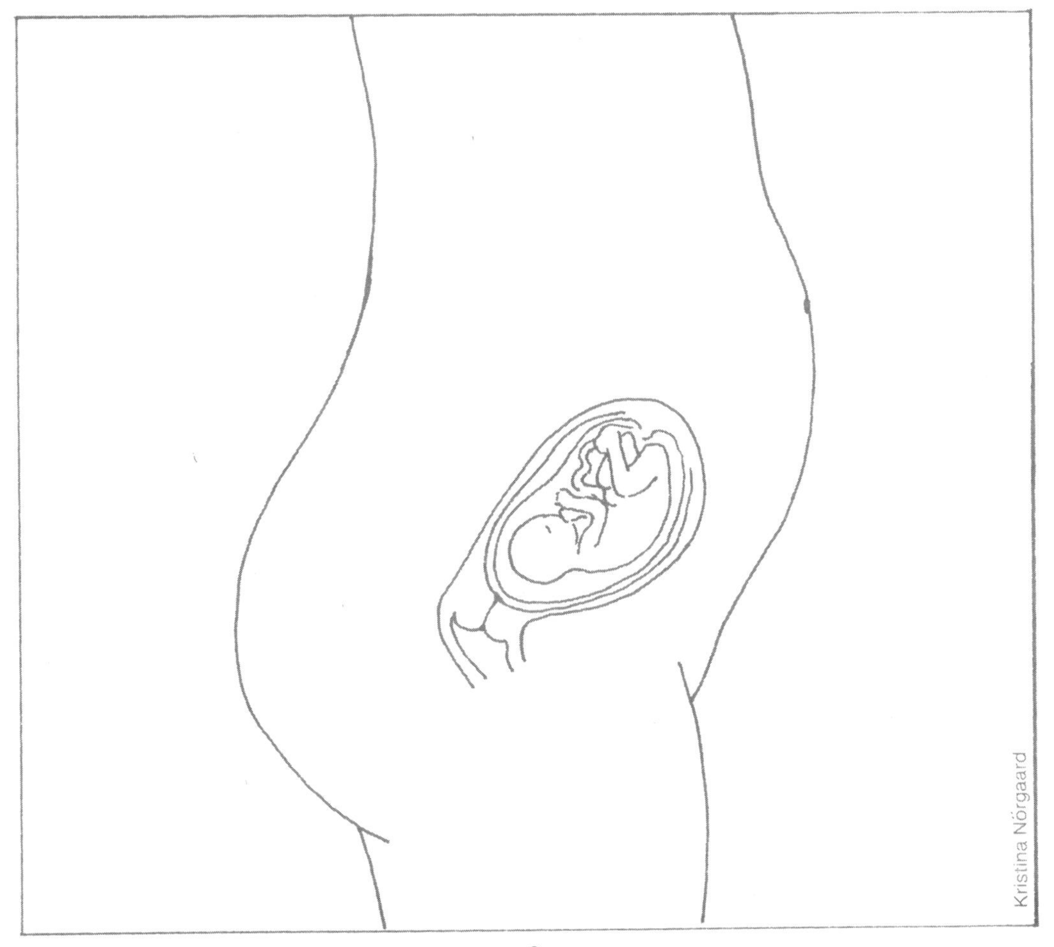

Fifth Month

During the fifth month, your baby weighs from a half to one pound and is about 10 to 12 inches long. Your baby is busy developing muscles and exercising them. Although he or she has been moving for some time now, it's during this month that most mothers feel the baby move for the first time. The time when you begin to feel your baby move is called "quickening."

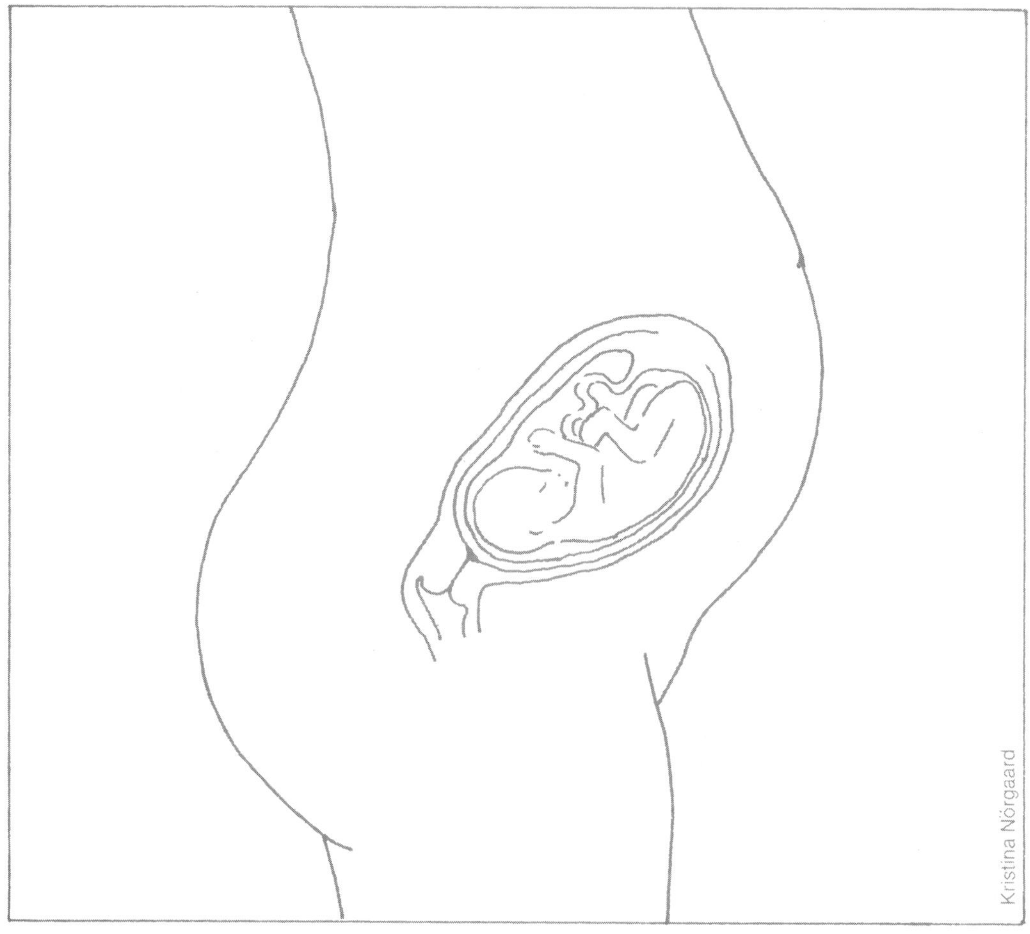

Sixth Month

At the end of the sixth month, your baby measures 11 to 14 inches long and may weigh as much as 1-1/2 to 2 pounds. The skin is reddish in color, wrinkled, and covered with a heavy, protective, creamy coating called vernix caseosa.

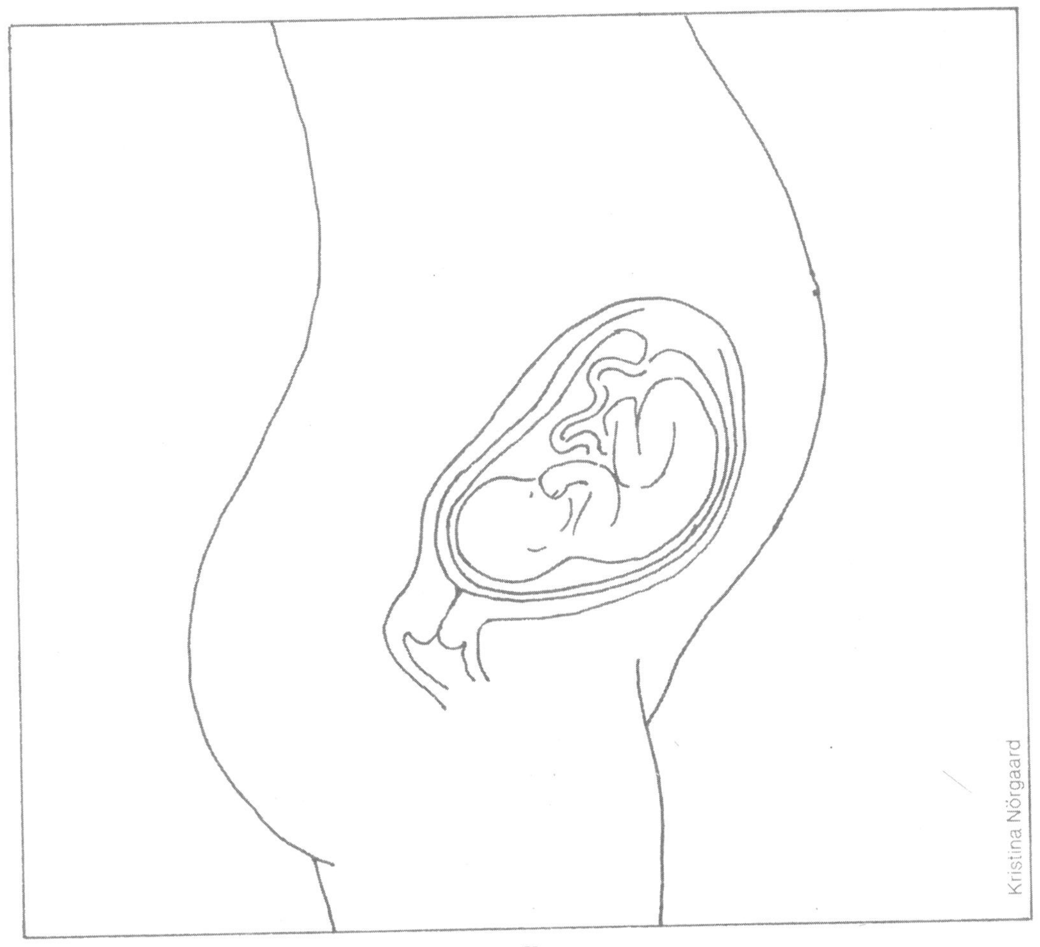

THE THIRD TRIMESTER

Seventh Month

During this month, your baby continues to grow and exercise. During the last part of the seventh month, a baby born prematurely has a chance for survival if skilled intensive care is provided.

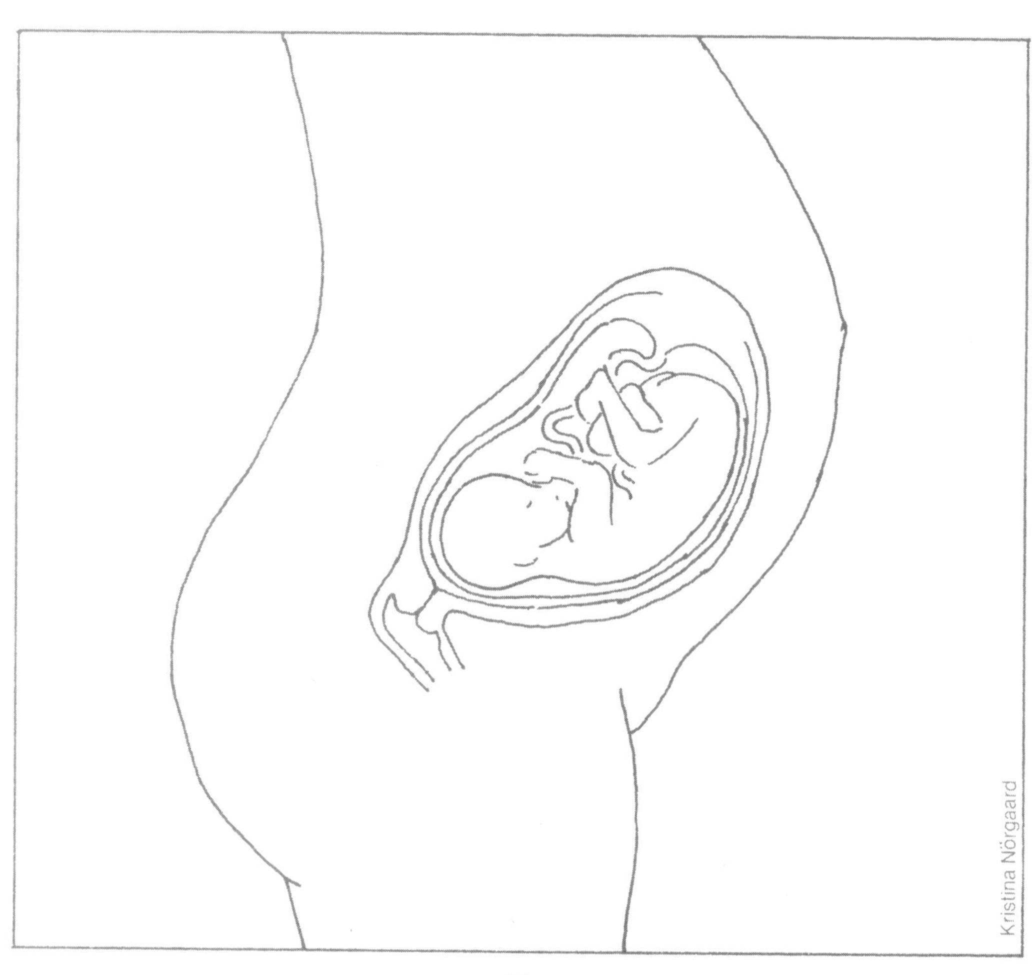

Eighth Month

Your baby is getting longer and fatter. He or she is now about 18 inches long with a weight of as much as five pounds. If born prematurely at the end of the eighth month, a baby's chances for survival are good.

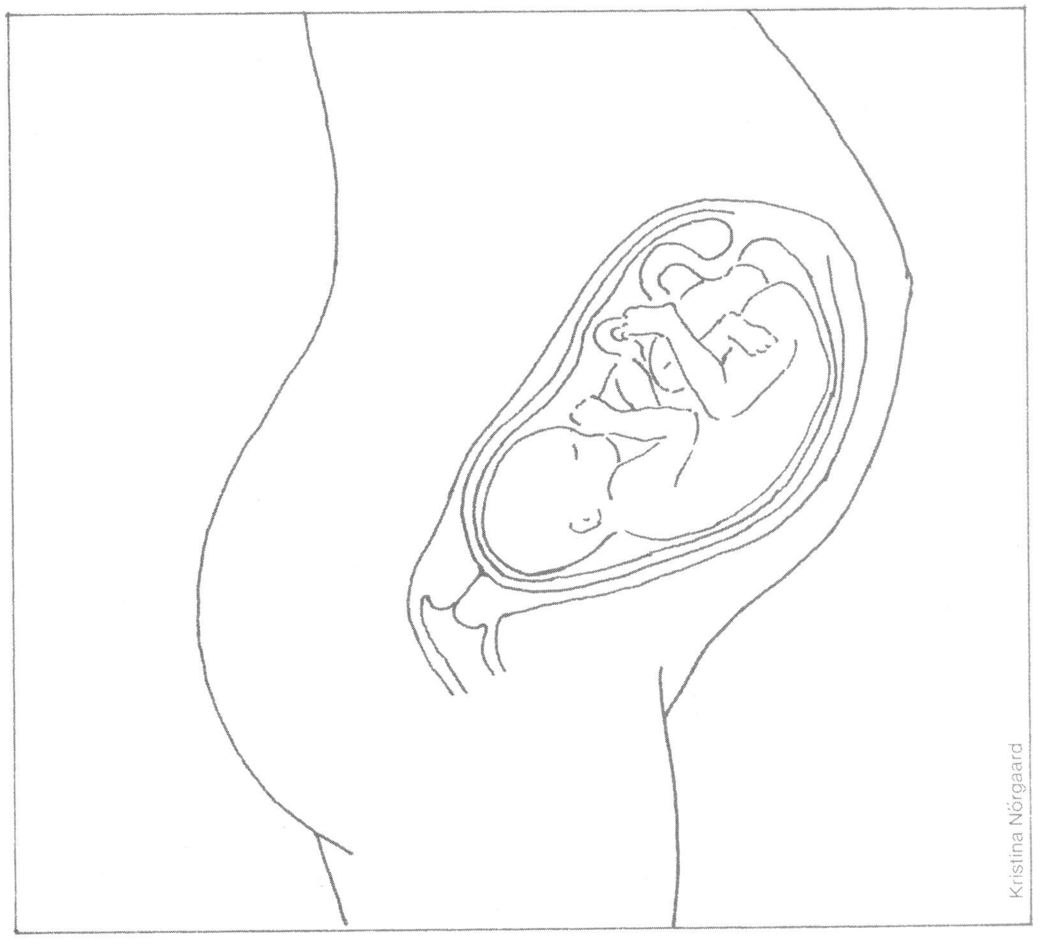

Ninth Month

During this month, your baby continues to grow and mature. At the end of the ninth month, an average full term baby weighs 7 to 7-1/2 pounds and is about 20 inches long. The skin is still coated with its creamy protective covering.

Some time during the ninth month your baby's position changes to get ready for labor and delivery. The baby drops down into your pelvis and the head engages in the birth position. Your baby is ready to be born.

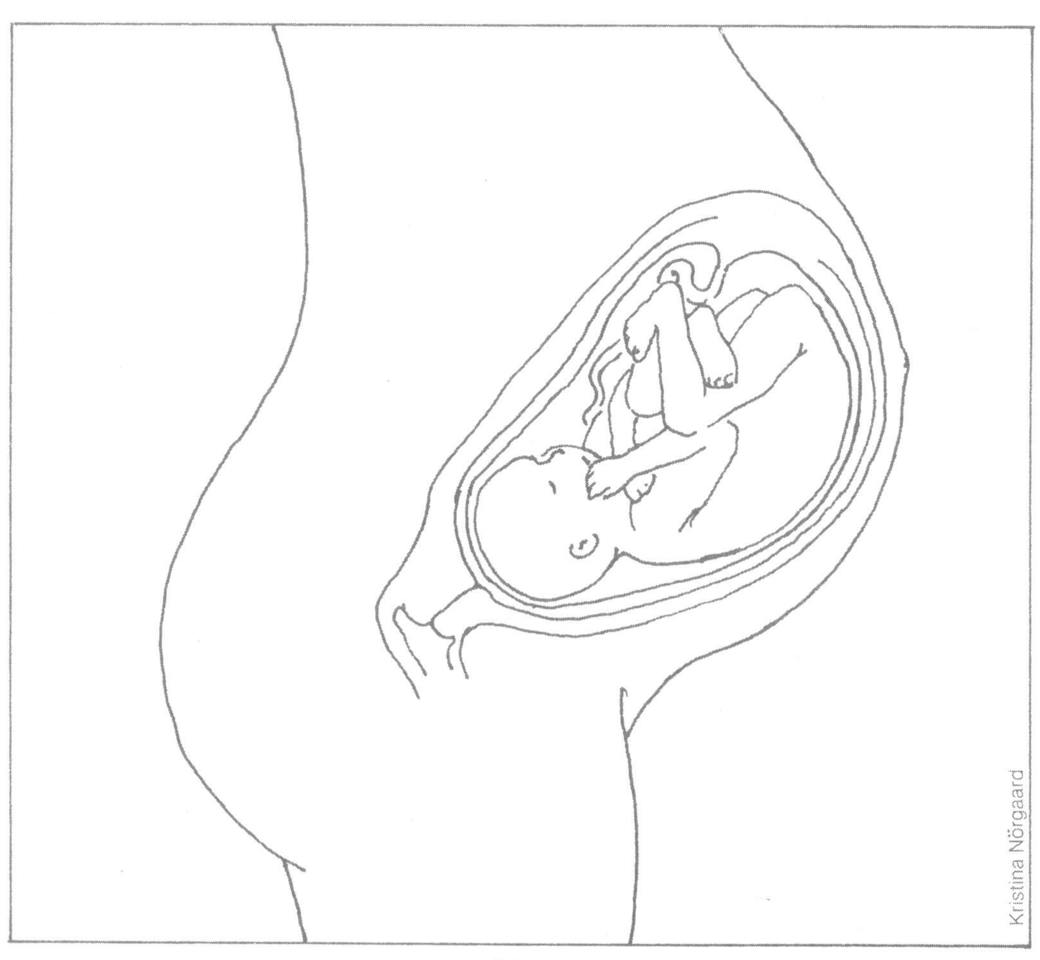

Section Two

COPING WITH BODILY CHANGES

Backache / Breasts (size and appearance) / Breasts (appearance of colostrum) / Constipation / Contractions (during pregnancy) / Faintness / Gums (bleeding and swelling) / Headaches / Heart Pounding / Heartburn or Intestinal Gas / Hemorrhoids / Muscle Cramps (especially in the legs) / Nausea and Vomiting (mild) / Nosebleeds / Pelvic Discomfort or Pain / Salivation (excessive) / Shortness of Breath / Skin (blotches and discoloring) / Stretch Marks / Swelling (feet, legs, and hands) / Tiredness / Vaginal Discharge / Varicose Veins

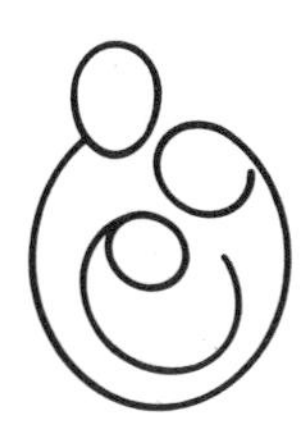

COPING WITH BODILY CHANGES

The following section describes some of the bodily changes that accompany pregnancy. Suggestions for coping comfortably with these changes are included. You may find some of these suggestions helpful. Remember, however, that no two pregnancies are exactly alike, and just because a particular problem is listed doesn't mean it will happen in your case. Few women will experience all of the discomforts mentioned, and you may avoid many or even most of them.

most likely at this time

may occur at this time

least likely at this time

BACKACHE

WHEN
mid to late pregnancy

1	2	3	4	5	6	7	8	9

WHY
As your body's weight, shape, and balance change, you may alter the way you sit or stand. This can cause muscle strain.

TRY THIS

- Make an effort to maintain good posture.
- Use sensible body mechanics. For example, squat instead of bending over. Rise from lying down by rolling on your side and pushing yourself up with your hands.
- Use a firm, flat mattress.
- Gentle daily exercise may help, especially for the sore spots. Try head rolling and shoulder rotating for discomfort in the upper back. Pelvic rocking should help the lower back. (See pages 26 to 30.)
- Wear comfortable shoes with heels of a height you are used to. This is not a good time for very high heels or an abrupt change to something different from what you usually wear.

BREASTS (changes in size and appearance)

WHEN
throughout pregnancy

1	2	3	4	5	6	7	8	9

WHY
Your breasts will increase in size because your milk glands enlarge and there is an increase in fatty tissue. They may become tender and more sensitive. As your blood supply increases and the blood vessels enlarge, bluish veins may appear.

TRY THIS

- Wear a supportive bra. This will ease strain on breast tissue and also on your back muscles if your breasts are heavy.
- Cotton allows the skin to breathe. Cotton bras are preferable to those made of synthetic fabrics. If you plan to nurse your baby, your nursing bras will probably be the same size or one cup size larger than those you need in late pregnancy.

BREASTS (appearance of colostrum)

WHEN
any time from fifth month on

1	2	3	4	5	6	7	8	9

WHY
Your breasts produce colostrum, which is a yellowish fluid, to be your baby's first food.

TRY THIS
- A cotton handkerchief or gauze pad tucked into each bra cup will absorb leaking fluid. Avoid plastic shields which trap moisture and cut off air circulation.

CONSTIPATION

WHEN
mid through late pregnancy

1	2	3	4	5	6	7	8	9

WHY
During pregnancy, your growing uterus takes up part of the working space of your digestive system, and hormones may also slow intestinal movement. Iron and vitamin supplements may also contribute to constipation in some cases.

TRY THIS
- Drink at least two quarts (8-10 glasses) of fluids daily. Try starting with a glass of fruit juice when you get up in the morning.
- Eat raw vegetables, fruits, and whole grains daily. Be sure to include prunes, dates, or figs in your diet.
- Try to give yourself time for a bowel movement at about the same time every day, or at least go when you have the urge. Don't put it off.
- Avoid mineral oil, which can remove Vitamins A, D, and E from your body. If you feel that you need a laxative, call the doctor. Don't take one on your own.

CONTRACTIONS (during pregnancy)

WHEN
You may feel them as early as four months. Most women don't notice them until seven or eight months.

1	2	3	4	5	6	7	8	9

WHY
Uterine muscles tighten irregularly from about four weeks of pregnancy on. These are called Braxton-Hicks contractions. They differ from the contractions of labor because they don't get stronger as time progresses, and they don't result in your baby's birth.

TRY THIS
- Continue your regular activities. Walking may be helpful.
- If you are uncomfortable, try to relax from head to toe. Understand and work with your body as it prepares in this normal way for labor and delivery.
- If contractions are severe or persistent, consult your doctor.

FAINTNESS

WHEN
early and late pregnancy

1	2	3	4	5	6	7	8	9

WHY
Low blood pressure, which can occur if you stand for long periods of time, may cause faintness. Faintness may also result from low blood sugar or too little iron in your blood (anemia).

TRY THIS
- When standing for long periods, move around frequently to stimulate your circulation.
- Especially during the last four or five months, try to give yourself frequent rest periods, even if they are very short.
- To keep your blood sugar up, eat healthful foods in small amounts at frequent intervals throughout the day.
- If anemia is detected during an office visit, changes in your diet may be suggested and iron pills may be advised.

GUMS (bleeding and swelling)

WHEN
mid to late pregnancy

1	2	3	4	5	6	7	8	9

WHY
During pregnancy, an increased supply of hormones, as well as the increase in your volume of circulation may cause tenderness, swelling, and bleeding of gums. A lack of vitamin C in your diet may also contribute to this condition.

TRY THIS
- Be sure that you don't neglect the program of attention your mouth requires, even though the tenderness of your gums might encourage you to forget about brushing.
- Vitamin C helps these tissues to be strong. It is best used by your body when it is taken as a natural part of your daily food.

HEADACHES

WHEN
throughout pregnancy

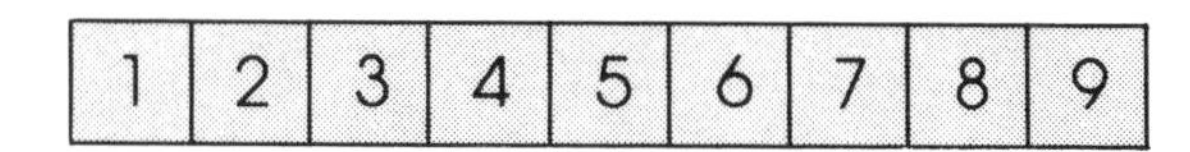

WHY
Nasal congestion, fatigue, eyestrain, anxiety, or tension are all possible causes of the headaches common to pregnancy.

TRY THIS
- For headaches of the sinus type, press a hot moist towel over your eyes and forehead.
- Relaxation and rest are often the most effective remedies for headaches.

- Because excessive doses of aspirin may be related to birth defects and problems during pregnancy, many physicians advise against any aspirin use during pregnancy and suggest a non-aspirin pain reliever. If your headaches persist or are severe, consult your doctor. Don't self medicate or continue to suffer.
- This is not the time to have new glasses or contact lenses fitted, and the lenses that were fine before your pregnancy might cause headache or strain now. Changes in vision may be related to your body's increased volume of circulation during your pregnancy, and you can be reassured that these problems are only temporary.

HEART POUNDING

WHEN
mid to late pregnancy

1	2	3	4	5	6	7	8	9

WHY
Occasional heart pounding is a normal response your body makes to meeting your baby's needs and the demands of your extra volume of circulation.

TRY THIS
- When you feel your heart pounding, consciously let go of tension all through your body. Sometimes it helps to start at your head and to relax each part of your body in turn until you reach your toes. (See page 30 for suggestions.)
- Breathe easily and comfortably.
- If heart pounding is a continuous problem, be sure to tell your doctor about it.

HEARTBURN OR INTESTINAL GAS

WHEN
mid to late pregnancy

1	2	3	4	5	6	7	8	9

WHY
During pregnancy, digestion may work more slowly. Your enlarging uterus crowds your stomach. Both of these things may lead to heartburn or intestinal gas.

TRY THIS
- To avoid crowding your stomach, eat several small nourishing meals daily, instead of three big ones. Relax, and eat slowly. Try to enjoy your meals.
- Avoid fried foods and others which tend to cause gas.
- Don't lie down directly after eating. When you do lie down, lie on your right side to help the stomach to empty.
- A very small amount of fatty food (butter or cream) eaten 15 to 30 minutes before a meal will stimulate digestion and cut down on stomach acid.
- Antacids and baking soda may cause you to hold fluid and may also bind B vitamins. If you feel you must take an antacid, try to take it at a time other than a meal.
- Use good posture. Give your stomach room to work.

HEMORRHOIDS

WHEN
mid to late pregnancy

1	2	3	4	5	6	7	8	9

WHY
The increased volume of your circulation causes dilation of veins in your rectum and vagina. There is added pressure from your growing uterus.

TRY THIS
- Try not to become constipated, as this will only make hemorrhoids more uncomfortable.
- Exercise the muscles around your vagina and anus (Kegel exercises). Tighten this part of your body, hold it for a few seconds, and then relax slowly. Do this at least 40 times a day. Try to work up to 100 or more. (See page 26 for suggestions.)
- Witch Hazel may be soothing. Soak a gauze square and hold it against the hemorrhoids for 20 minutes while you rest lying down. Lie on your left side, and rest your upper arm and leg on pillows.

MORNING SICKNESS (See Nausea and Vomiting)

MUSCLE CRAMPS (especially in the legs)

WHEN
mid to late pregnancy

1	2	3	4	5	6	7	8	9

WHY
Calcium, which affects muscle contractions, is less easily absorbed during pregnancy. Pressure from your growing uterus slows circulation in the legs. This may lead to cramps.

TRY THIS
- Watch your diet. Be sure to eat foods which contain plenty of calcium.
- When taking calcium pills, eat foods which contain calcium at the same time. Calcium is best used by your body when it is in the presence of other nutrients found around it naturally.
- To ease a cramp in your calf, push away from your body with your heel. At the same time, pull your toes toward your shoulder. This helps stretch the muscle out of its cramp.
- Gentle massage or a hot water bottle on the cramp may help.
- Avoid lying on your back. The weight of your body on major blood vessels will slow circulation to the legs and increase the likelihood of cramps. Lie on your left side instead.

NAUSEA AND VOMITING (mild)

WHEN
first three months

1	2	3	4	5	6	7	8	9

WHY
Your body may be reacting to the hormones of pregnancy. Too little Vitamin B_6 or too little glycogen, the natural sugar stored in your liver, can cause nausea. Emotions are another possible cause of nausea during pregnancy.

TRY THIS

- Nausea is especially bothersome on an empty stomach, so you might try a protein snack such as lean meat or cheese before going to bed. (Protein takes longer to digest.)
- If you are especially troubled by nausea in the morning, nibble on some crackers before you get out of bed.
- Eat small but frequent meals during the day. Eat slowly and try to stay relaxed.
- Drink fruit juice at the end of breakfast.
- Extra Vitamin B_6 might help.

NOSEBLEEDS

WHEN
throughout pregnancy

1	2	3	4	5	6	7	8	9

WHY
Membranes become overloaded during pregnancy from the increased volume of circulation. This causes nosebleeds in some women.

TRY THIS

- Be sure you are getting enough Vitamin C. This vitamin promotes strong tissues.
- During a nosebleed, lie down and apply cold compresses to your nose.
- A higher level of humidity will help decrease the risk of nosebleeds. Try a humidifier if the air in your home tends to be very dry.
- Try a thin coating of Vaseline in each nostril, especially at bedtime.

PELVIC DISCOMFORT OR PAIN

WHEN
mid to late pregnancy

1	2	3	4	5	6	7	8	9

WHY
During pregnancy, the pubic bone and sacroiliac joints relax to increase the size and flexibility of available space for the birth canal. This may cause pressure on the sciatic nerve, with pain in the pelvic area and down the thigh and into the leg.

TRY THIS

- A heating pad may bring some relief.
- Some women find massage helpful.
- Experiment with different positions to find the one that's most comfortable. Try sleeping on your side, with one leg forward and the other back as if you were running.

SALIVATION (excessive)

WHEN
mid to late pregnancy

1	2	3	4	5	6	7	8	9

WHY

During pregnancy, the salivary glands increase production. In a few women this increase may become excessive. We are not exactly sure why this is so.

TRY THIS

- Chewing gum may help keep excessive salivation under control.
- Sometimes eating several small meals instead of three large ones during the day will help with this problem.

SHORTNESS OF BREATH

WHEN

mid to late pregnancy
in the ninth month, after your baby drops, you may find some relief

1	2	3	4	5	6	7	8	9

WHY

Your growing uterus takes up part of your breathing space. It causes pressure on your diaphragm.

TRY THIS

- Hold your arms up over your head. This raises your rib cage and temporarily gives you more breathing space.
- Try sleeping with pillows propped to keep you in a position that makes breathing easier.
- Practice very slow, deep breathing while you are very relaxed. Try this every day. It will help you use your lung space to its greatest capacity.
- Try lying on your left side.

SKIN (blotches and discoloring)

WHEN

mid to late pregnancy

1	2	3	4	5	6	7	8	9

WHY

Extra deposits of pigment are triggered by a hormone which increases during pregnancy. This may cause brown coloring over cheeks, nose, and forehead, as well as on the nipples and in a line from the naval to the pubic bone.

TRY THIS

- Avoid sunburn, which may deepen skin coloring.
- Be reassured that the hormone which causes these discolorations will decrease after your baby is born, and the spots will disappear of their own accord.

STRETCH MARKS

WHEN

mid to late pregnancy

1	2	3	4	5	6	7	8	9

WHY

About 90% of pregnant women experience stretch marks to some degree. Stretch marks are a type of scar tissue which forms when the skin's normal elasticity is not sufficient to accommodate the stretching required during pregnancy. Stretch marks occur most frequently on the abdomen, but some women also get them on the thighs and breasts.

TRY THIS

- Be sure that your diet contains sufficient protein. This will help you keep healthy skin.
- Vitamin E and Vitamin C may be helpful, so be sure that your diet includes these nutrients.
- Keeping your skin soft and supple won't prevent stretch marks, but it may help minimize them. Try a gentle massage with oil or cream. Some women find that cocoa butter helps keep the skin soft.
- Although stretch marks may not disappear after delivery, those that remain usually fade into a light silvery color.

SWELLING (feet, legs, and hands)

WHEN

mid to late pregnancy

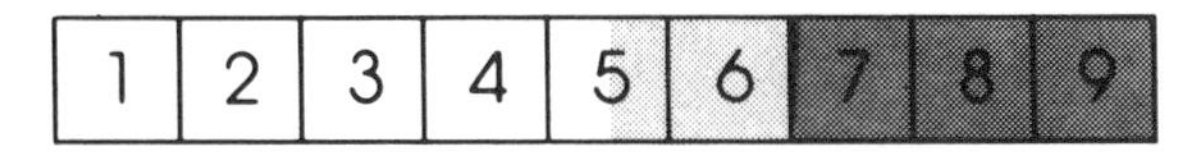

WHY

Your body naturally holds water during pregnancy. The growing uterus puts pressure on blood vessels which return fluid from the legs. Tight clothing, especially around the ankles, legs, and lower body can increase swelling by slowing down circulation. Long periods of standing or sitting can slow down circulation in the legs. Too little protein in your diet may also cause your body to retain fluid.

TRY THIS

- Wear loose clothing. Be sure to avoid tight pants, waist bands, knee or ankle socks.
- Don't remain on your feet for long periods of time. Try to sit down frequently with your legs raised at a mild angle to your body. Try to avoid sitting with your feet on the floor for lengthy periods. Don't sit with your legs crossed, because this can interfere with circulation.
- Be sure to keep your daily diet rich in protein.
- Drinking clear fluids (water) will help pull the extra fluid out of your system.

TIREDNESS

WHEN

early and late pregnancy

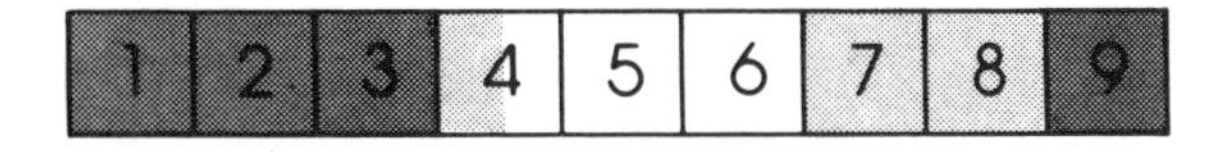

WHY

Fatigue is a natural effect of hormones of pregnancy. Extra energy is needed to carry and care for your developing baby. Tiredness may also result from anemia, which is not uncommon during pregnancy. Inadequate iron in the diet is frequently the cause of anemia.

TRY THIS

- Early to bed, late to rise, with rest periods during the day as well.

- Balance the rest with daily exercise. (Walking is excellent.) Exercise stimulates circulation and brings energized oxygen and nutrition to your entire body.
- Have your doctor check for anemia. If anemia is a problem for you, changes in diet and/or iron supplements may be suggested.

VAGINAL DISCHARGE

WHEN
throughout pregnancy

1	2	3	4	5	6	7	8	9

WHY
Increased blood supply and hormones cause your vagina to increase its normal secretions. The normal acidic atmosphere changes too, creating a more fertile setting for the common vaginal infection, monilia.

TRY THIS
- Wear skirts rather than slacks, and underwear with cotton crotch. Air circulation will help.
- Avoid douching during pregnancy because it is possible at this time to introduce air into your circulatory system or, in the last months, to break your bag of waters. If it is medically necessary for you to douche, your doctor or nurse midwife will explain exactly how you should do it.
- Call your doctor or nurse midwife if your discharge burns, itches, smells bad, or causes your genitals to become swollen.
- Be alert to the signs of pre-term labor. (See page 80.) Call your doctor or nurse midwife to report an increase or change in vaginal discharge, especially if the discharge is clear and watery or tinged with blood.

VARICOSE VEINS

WHEN
mid to late pregnancy

1	2	3	4	5	6	7	8	9

WHY
Veins in your legs can become overloaded as a result of slowed circulation from a greater quantity of blood, and also from the pressure of your growing uterus.

TRY THIS
- Avoid standing for long periods. If you must stand, try to move about.
- Rest several times a day with your legs raised at a mild angle to your body.
- Leg exercises will help your blood to circulate better.
- Elastic stockings may help. They must be put on before getting out of bed, while your legs are relatively free of the extra blood which overloads them when you stand.

Section Three

KEEPING HEALTHY AND FIT

Exercises While Waiting

Good Nutrition Is Important

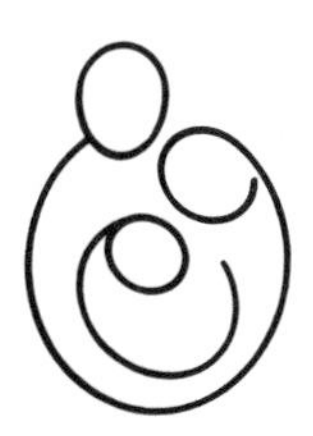

EXERCISES WHILE WAITING

The following pages contain exercises designed to improve posture, strengthen important muscles, relieve tension and pressure, and help you relax. These exercises will help you to feel more comfortable during your pregnancy as well as prepare your body for labor and delivery. Many of them will be useful during your postpartum days as you work to restore your body to its pre-pregnancy fitness.

Begin each of these exercises gradually – twice will do for each exercise the first time around. Work up to five, or even ten, but do it gradually. Remember to keep within the bounds of what is comfortable for you. If a particular exercise causes you discomfort or pain, stop. After the fifth month of pregnancy, exercises done on the back may be inadvisable. Ask your physician if there are any special cautions you should observe at this time.

If more than one exercise is suggested for the same purpose, you don't have to do them all. Pick one that suits you best, or alternate for variety. The important thing is to do what makes sense for you.

PELVIC FLOOR EXERCISES

These are perhaps the most important exercises you can do to prepare your body for labor and delivery and for a rapid postpartum recovery. A strong and elastic pelvic floor can reduce or prevent problems such as sagging organs or leaking urine. Because these exercises strengthen the muscles used in intercourse and orgasm, they may also increase sexual enjoyment.

Pelvic floor exercises are easily and conveniently done almost anytime or anywhere. Try them while you're in a car or train, watching TV, brushing your teeth, talking on the telephone, doing things around the house, waiting around, making love, or just doing nothing. You'll find these exercises very helpful in promoting healing and restoring muscle tone after your baby is born.

KEGEL EXERCISE #1

You can do this exercise in any position — lying down, sitting, or standing. Your legs should be slightly apart.

Tighten and then release the muscles around your vagina. Work up to doing this 100 or more times a day. (Note that 20 times 5, or 10 times 10 will be more effective and less tiring than 100 times without stopping.)

Here are two techniques to help you get the feel of this exercise.

(1) Place your hand over your pubic bones. Imagine you are trying to contract your vaginal muscles as far up as your hand.

(2) Try this exercise while urinating. If you can start and stop the flow or urine at will, you've got it.

KEGEL EXERCISE #2

Tighten and release the vaginal muscles as in Kegel #1. This time however, you will do it more slowly. Tighten the muscles slowly as you count to six (or time yourself using a clock with a second hand). Then slowly relax to a count of four. Then tighten and hold again for six seconds. Relax for four. Begin with a minute. Work up to five minutes at a time, several times a day. Breathe normally as you do this exercise. Resist the temptation to hold your breath as you count.

BETTER POSTURE AND COMFORT

Here are simple exercises to improve your posture while sitting and standing. You will look better and feel more comfortable if you have good posture. Skip the tailor sitting exercises if they cause pain in the pubic bone area. You may already have separation here, and in that case you shouldn't continue this particular set of exercises.

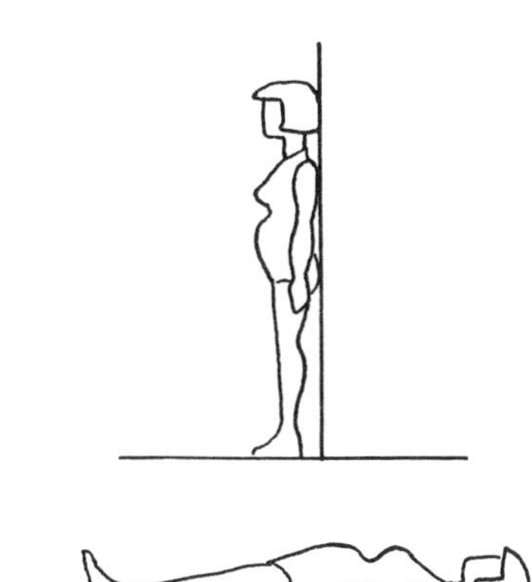

BACK FLATTENING #1

Stand with your back to the wall and your feet a few inches away. Your head, shoulders, and buttocks should be touching the wall. Stand tall and straighten your neck and your lower back muscles. Count to ten. Relax. Do it again. Work up to ten times.

BACK FLATTENING #2

Lie on the floor on your back, with your toes pointing up. Straighten your back and pretend you are trying to push yourself — still flat on your back — straight through the floorboards. Count to ten. Relax. Do it again. Work up to ten times.

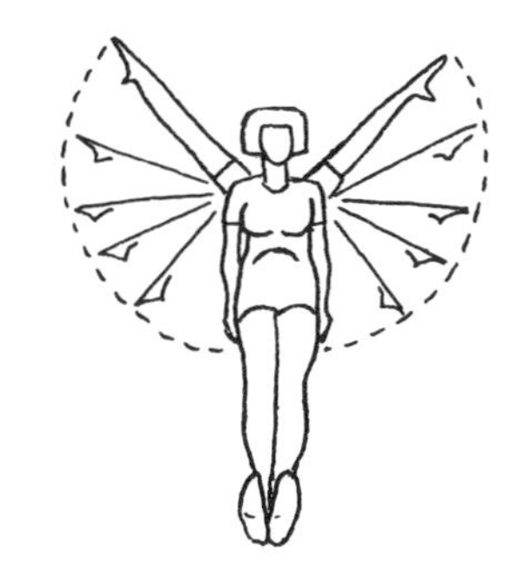

BACK FLATTENING #3

Lie on the floor on your back as in exercise #2. Keeping your arms straight and on the floor at all times, raise your hands until your arms are straight above your head. Then bring them slowly back to your sides. (Some of us learned the movements for this exercise as children playing "Angels in the Snow.") Repeat ten times.

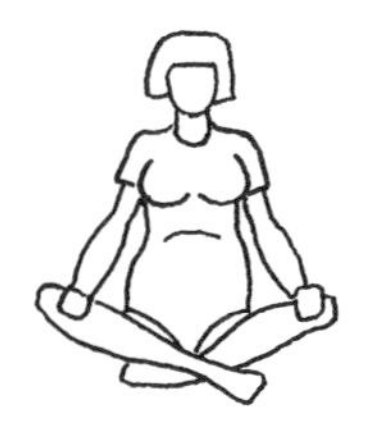

TAILOR SITTING #1

Sit on the floor with your legs crossed just over the ankles. Your back should be slightly rounded. This position will help to stretch the muscles of your inner thighs and get you used to relaxing your pelvic floor with your legs apart. Try sitting in this position while reading or watching TV.

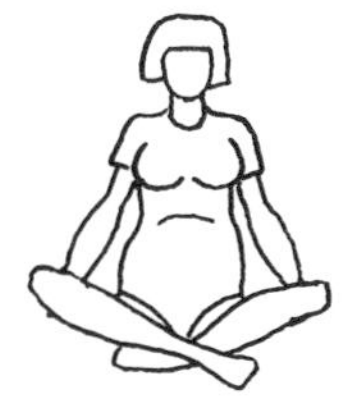

TAILOR SITTING #2

While sitting in the tailor position, hold your hands one under each knee. Press your knees to the floor while providing pressure in the other direction with your hands.

TAILOR SITTING #3

Sit on the floor with the soles of your feet together. Slowly pull your heels as close to your body as you can comfortably.

EXERCISES FOR LEGS

These two exercises will help relieve circulatory problems in your legs. They are useful for dealing with discomfort from swelling, varicose veins, and cramps.

SWINGING FEET

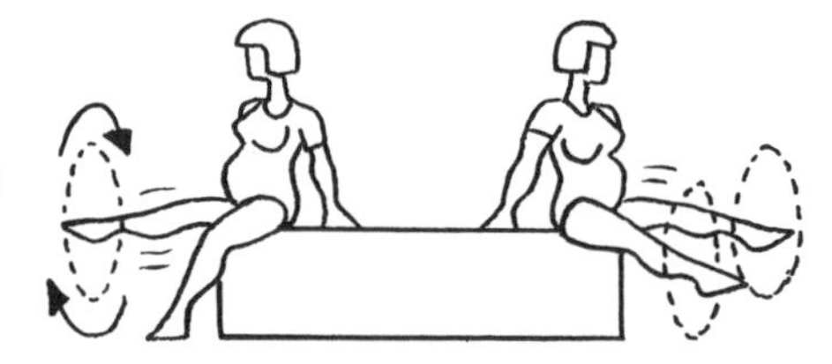

Draw large circles in the air with your toes. You can do both feet at once, or one foot at a time. Do some circles from left to right and some from right to left.

LEG LIFTS

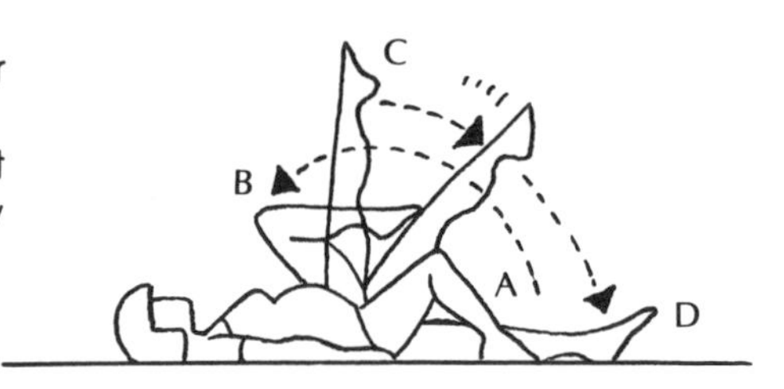

Lie on your back with bent knees and your feet flat on the floor. One leg at a time, pull your knee up toward your shoulder. Then straighten your leg and point it toward the ceiling. Without bending your leg, lower it smoothly and gently to the floor. Return to your starting position. Repeat with the other leg. Do not try to do this exercise with both legs at once.

EXERCISES FOR UPPER BACK

These exercises will help prevent and relieve aches and tension in the neck, upper back, and shoulders.

ARM STRETCH

Stand up and keep your feet flat on the floor. Stretch one arm at a time, reaching as high as you can. Stretch one arm and then the other. Work up to ten or more times.

BACK STRETCH

Lie flat on your back on the floor. Point your toes to the ceiling. Stretch first one side and then the other. Pull your toes up toward your shoulders and push away with your heels. Work up to ten or more times.

HEAD ROLLING

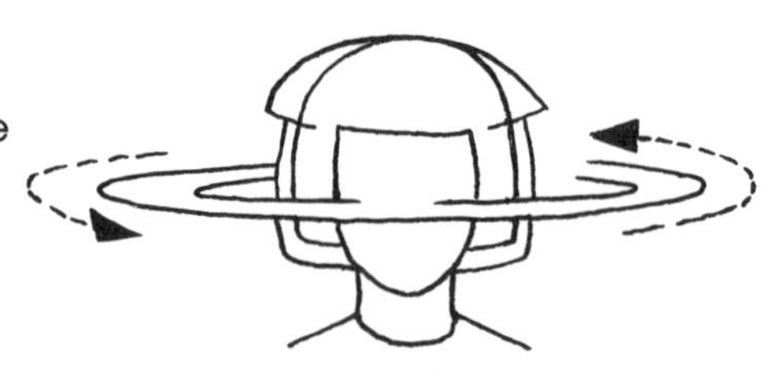

You can sit on a chair or the edge of a bed for this exercise. Or, if you prefer, try sitting on the floor in the tailor position. Relax your neck and shoulder muscles. Roll your head around and around. Work up to five times clockwise and five times counterclockwise. Be sure to keep your neck as relaxed as possible, and let the weight of your head roll it around.

SHOULDER ROTATION #1

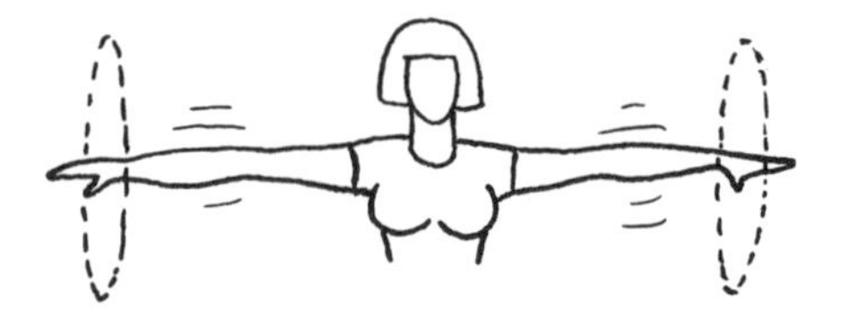

Extend your arms straight out from your shoulders. Make circles with your arms. Do five in one direction and five in the other. Stretch your arms way out straight and feel the muscles in your shoulder blades as they work.

SHOULDER ROTATION #2

Put one hand on each shoulder and point your elbows straight out from your sides. Make circles with your elbows just as you did with your arms straight in the previous exercise. Both shoulder rotation exercises can be done while sitting in the tailor position.

EXERCISES FOR ABDOMINAL MUSCLES

Before doing the exercises to strengthen your abdominal muscles, follow the procedures suggested below to check for separation of these muscles. If your muscles have separated, you should do the exercise designed to prevent further separation. If not, you can safely go on to the more strenuous exercises that follow.

Separation Check

Your abdominal muscles are arranged in two bands. During pregnancy, these muscles may separate at the seam. Here's how to check for separation. Lie on your back. (You need your clothes off for this one.) Bend your knees and keep your feet flat on the floor. Raise your head and shoulders slowly until your neck is about eight inches off the floor. If you can see a hollow (in early pregnancy or postpartum) or a bulge (in late pregnancy) your abdominal muscles are weak. Do the exercise that follows to help avoid further separation.

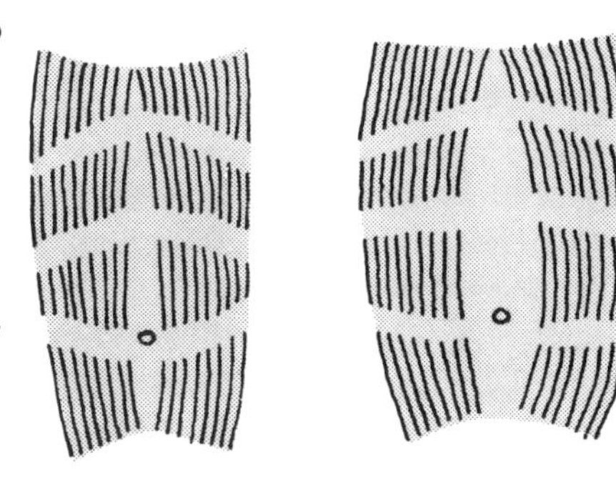

Exercise for Separated Muscles

Lie on your back with your knees bent and your feet flat on the floor. Cross your hands and place them on your abdomen. Push the sides of your abdomen toward the center. Raise your head as you did in the separation check, but this time stop just before the point where you would see the hollow or the bulge. Work up to doing this at least five times, twice a day.

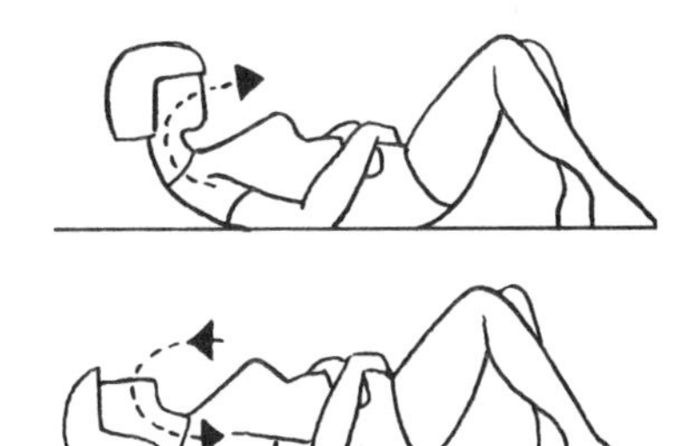

Back Rounding

If you begin this exercise early in your pregnancy, you'll probably find it helpful. It's a difficult one to begin later on, however, so if you have trouble, skip it. Do not use this exercise if your abdominal muscles have separated.

Lie on your back with bent knees and your feet flat on the floor. Rest your chin on your chest. Reach for your knees with your hands. As you exhale slowly, raise your head and shoulders as far as you can with your waist still on the floor. Work up to five times, twice a day.

BREATHE IN, BREATHE OUT, AND BLOW

Lie on your back with your feet flat on the floor and your knees bent. Put a pillow under your head if you wish. Breathe in through your nose and let your abdomen rise gently. Breathe out through your nose and let your abdomen return to its normal position. Now, without taking another breath, blow out gently through your mouth as long as you can. You should feel your abdominal muscles tighten. Work up to doing this ten times.

PELVIC ROCK #1

Get down on your hands and knees. Keep your knees a little bit apart and your back flat. Your hands should be directly under your shoulders, not farther forward or back. Tighten up your buttock muscles and pull your hips in toward your chin. At the same time, tighten your abdominal muscles and arch your back like an angry cat. Work up to ten times or more.

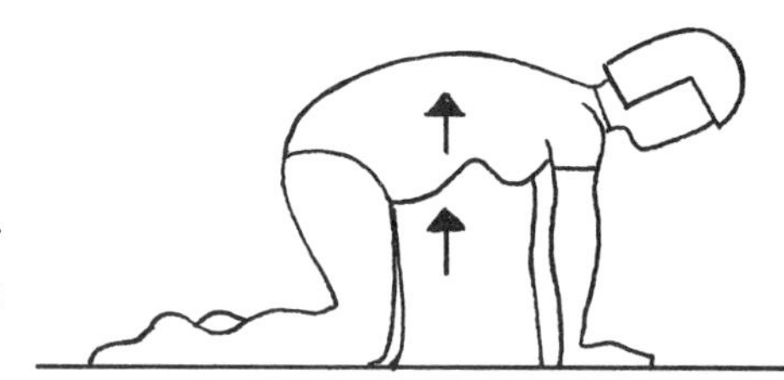

PELVIC ROCK #2

Lie on the floor with your knees bent and the soles of your feet flat on the floor. Flatten your back to the floor while at the same time pulling in your abdominal muscles. Be sure to keep your buttocks on the floor while you are pushing down with your back. Work up to ten times or more.

RELAXING TECHNIQUES

Knowing how to relax completely is something you will find very useful when you are anxious or physically uncomfortable. The kind of relaxing we are talking about is not simply the absence of activity. It is a conscious release of tension as you concentrate on one part of your body after another. To learn to do this requires practice, and it may help if you do your relaxing as a regular part of your exercise routine.

RELAXING #1

Choose a position that is comfortable for you. You may sit, stand, or lie down. Let go of tension starting at the top of your head. Concentrate on one part of your body after another in turn until you reach your feet. Take as long as you need and breathe naturally. For variety, you can begin at your toes and work up. Follow this with Relaxing #2 below.

RELAXING #2

Here's a short cut to relaxing your body. Concentrate on and relax each of these four areas in turn:

(1) face, neck, and shoulders
(2) hands
(3) bottom and thighs
(4) feet

When you need to relax in a hurry, this shortcut to total relaxation may help you.

GOOD NUTRITION IS IMPORTANT

What you eat or don't eat during your pregnancy really does make a difference to your developing baby as well as to your own health and comfort. Although many people believe that an unborn child can draw needed nourishment from the mother's body even if she eats poorly, we now know that isn't so. If your diet lacks essential nutrients, your baby will suffer the effects along with you.

At one time, it was thought that the placenta served as a barrier to protect the fetus from harmful substances taken by the mother. This is not so either. Virtually everything a pregnant woman eats or drinks will reach her baby in some way.

The effects of poor nutrition are passed from one generation to the next. What your mother ate before you were born, what you ate throughout your growing years, as well as your present diet all influence your unborn child.

If in the past your diet was inadequate for any reason, of course it's impossible to go back and do things over again. NOW is the time, if you haven't already begun, to start planning your meals carefully so that you and your baby will be well nourished.

PLANNING YOUR DIET

You don't have to read this section from start to finish or become a walking nutrition textbook in order to plan nourishing meals. Here are some guidelines that will help you use this material in the way that's best for you.

(1) Be sure to look at the chart on page 33. This tells you the recommended daily quantity you need of protein, vitamins, and minerals. Use this chart as a reference.

(2) Pages 37 to 43 describe in greater detail the various substances you need. Read this section only if you want to understand why you should do certain things.

(3) Skim the section on food additives, pages 44 to 45. Begin to look for these items on product labels as you shop. Avoid them.

(4) For information on supplemental vitamins, fluid intake, and vegetarian diets, see pages 43, 45, 46.

(5) Page 36 provides an alternate approach to diet planning. The major food groups are listed along with reasons to include them, and serving quantities. Some people find this chart helpful in planning their meals.

(6) Use pages 34 to 35 to do your own diet diagnosis.

- What you eat directly affects how your baby grows.
- If you eat or drink harmful things, the placenta cannot keep them away from your baby.
- The effects of poor nutrition are passed from one generation to the next.
- You can begin NOW to build a healthier future for both you and your baby.

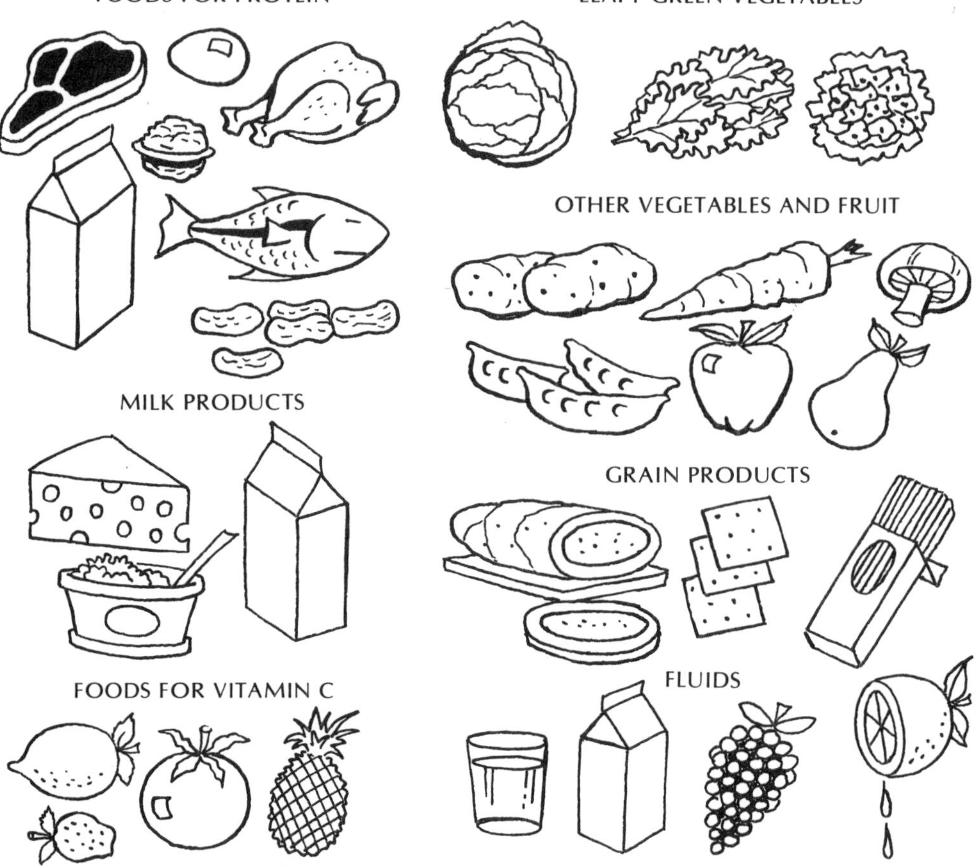

DAILY DIET ESSENTIALS FOR PREGNANT WOMEN

The chart on the next page tells how much of the various food substances you will need each day. Column Two lists the lowest possible amount you could probably make do with. It is provided for your information only, and should not be the guideline you use in meal planning. Column Four lists the upper limits generally considered safe for each of these substances. In special cases, however, your doctor may modify this list.

Columns One and Three provide the quantities generally recommended during pregnancy. Use these columns as your guide unless your doctor tells you otherwise. Note that certain of the recommendations differ slightly. We've included both to show you that even experts disagree, and that you shouldn't worry over small differences. To be on the safe side, many women aim for the larger of the two quantities recommended.

The labels on many food products tell you the quantity of various vitamins and minerals, protein and carbohydrates, as well as the calorie count you will find in a serving of that product. Use this information in conjunction with the guidelines on this chart.

You might find this chart easier to use if you circle in green the guidelines you will use. If your doctor makes any changes for you, write in the new numbers in green as well.

DAILY DIET ESSENTIALS FOR PREGNANT WOMEN

	Recommended** Dietary Allowance (RDA)	LOWER* LIMIT	U.S. Recommended* Daily Allowances (U.S. RDAs)	UPPER* LIMIT
CALORIES	2400			
PROTEIN	70-80 grams			
FAT SOLUBLE VITAMINS				
Vitamin A	5000 I.U.	5000 I.U.	8000 I.U.	8000 I.U.
Vitamin D	400 I.U.	400 I.U.	400 I.U.	400 I.U.
Vitamin E	15 I.U.	30 I.U.	30 I.U.	60 I.U.
WATER SOLUBLE VITAMINS				
Vitamin C	60 mg.	60 mg.	60 mg.	120 mg.
B Complex:				
Folic Acid	800 mcg.	400 mcg.	800 mcg.	800 mcg.
Thiamine (B_1)	1.3 mg.	1.5 mg.	1.7 mg.	3 mg.
Riboflavin (B_2)	1.7 mg.	1.7 mg.	2 mg.	3.4 mg.
Niacin (B_3)	15 mg.	20 mg.	20 mg.	40 mg.
Pyridoxine (B_6)	2.5 mg.	2 mg.	2.5 mg.	4 mg.
Vitamin B_{12}	4 mcg.	6 mcg.	8 mcg.	12 mcg.
Biotin		300 mcg.	300 mcg.	600 mcg.
Pantothenic Acid		10 mg.	10 mg.	20 mg.
MINERALS				
Calcium	1200 mg.	125 mg.	1300 mg.	2000 mg.
Phosphorus (Optional — must not exceed calcium level)	1200 mg.	125 mg.	1300 mg.	2000 mg.
Iodine	.125 mg.	.15 mg.	.15 mg.	.3 mg.
Iron	36 mg.	18 mg.	18 mg.	60 mg.
Magnesium	450 mg.	100 mg.	450 mg.	800 mg.
Copper		1 mg.	2 mg.	4 mg.
Zinc	20 mg.	7.5 mg.	15 mg.	30 mg.

*U.S. Recommended Daily Allowances for Pregnant or Lactating Women. U.S. Food and Drug Administration, 1978.

**Recommended Daily Dietary Allowances for Pregnant Women. Food and Nutrition Board, National Research Council, National Academy of Sciences. Revised 1974.

PERSONAL DIET DIAGNOSIS

Use this chart to help you diagnose the adequacy of your own diet. For three days or more, write down everything you eat or drink. Do what you would normally do during this time. Don't change your eating habits just because you are writing things down. At the end of each day, add up the quantities in each column. Compare what you have done with what you should have done. Circle in red any items that should be omitted or decreased. Circle in green any items that should be increased. Write in using green any items that should be added. Note the reasons for each of these changes at the right. This will help you remember.

Food	Amt.	Calories	Protein gms.	Calcium mgs.	Vitamins	Iron	Sodium	OK ?	Change Because

Food	Amt.	Calories	Protein gms.	Calcium mgs.	Vitamins	Iron	Sodium	OK ?	Change Because

NUTRITION PLAN...WHILE WAITING

WHAT?	WHY?	HOW MUCH?
FOODS FOR PROTEIN meat, fish, liver, poultry, eggs, milk, soybeans, nuts, peanut butter	Protein is the building material for all body tissues. It supplies energy and promotes healthy growth and development.	Four servings or more per day. A serving consists of 3 oz. of fish, poultry, or lean meat (cooked); 2 large eggs; 3/4 cup cooked soybeans.
MILK PRODUCTS milk, buttermilk, yogurt, cheese, cottage cheese	Milk products are an excellent source of vitamins, minerals, and protein. They are the best utilized source of calcium, which helps build strong bones and teeth.	Four servings (or equivalent sources of protein and calcium) per day. You may count milk products used in preparing soups, custards, or puddings in your total.
FOODS FOR VITAMIN C citrus fruits, strawberries, pine-apples, tomatoes, peppers	Vitamin C is needed to build strong body cells and blood. Healthy gums, teeth, and bones require it.	At least one serving per day. Your body can't store Vitamin C, so be sure to eat something from this group at least once in a day.
LEAFY GREEN VEGETABLES spinach, broccoli, brussels sprouts, collard greens, kale, cabbage, etc.	These are a source of Vitamin A. They are needed for proper development of your baby's bones, hair, skin, and glands. They aid development of the eyes, and are necessary for good vision.	Two servings per day. A serving is 3/4 cup cooked, or 1 cup raw.
OTHER VEGETABLES AND FRUIT potatoes, carrots, yams, bean sprouts, squash, mushrooms, pea pods, apples, peaches, pears, apricots, plums, grapes, berries, prunes, dates, figs, raisins	Yellow vegetables and fruits are a source of Vitamin A. A number of different minerals are found in the foods in this group.	One serving per day. Raw carrots are a good snack. Try a piece of fresh fruit or dried fruit such as raisins.
GRAIN PRODUCTS bread, cereal, crackers, pastas, rice, wheat germ, tortillas, grits.	Whole grain products contain B Vitamins. Avoid highly processed grains which have lost much of their nutritional value and simply add calories.	Three or more servings per day. One serving is a slice of bread or a half cup of a cooked grain product like cereal or pasta.
FLUIDS water, milk, fruit juice, herb teas	An adequate supply of liquids is necessary to keep your body systems functioning well during pregnancy.	Two quarts (8-10) glasses per day.

CARBOHYDRATES

Carbohydrates (starches and sugars) are necessary in your diet, but many people consume far more than they require. It's unlikely that you will have to concern yourself with carbohydrate intake except to make sure that you don't overdo it. A food high in carbohydrates and little else can be a quick source of energy, but it will also be a quick source of calories and unneeded weight gain. If you concentrate on meeting protein, vitamin, and mineral requirements, your diet will probably contain the carbohydrates you need without any special effort.

PROTEINS

Proteins are complex chemicals which have two important functions. First, they serve as the building materials of body tissue. From your hair to your toenails, most of your body — your blood, bones, muscles, and other tissues — are made up primarily of proteins. The second function of proteins is to act as enzymes which regulate the chemical reactions that keep a body growing and functioning.

When you understand what two roles proteins play, it's easy to see how very important an adequate supply would be for an unborn child. The developing baby is building new tissue and experiencing chemical reactions at a very rapid rate. Proteins are vital to these processes.

Too little protein in a pregnant woman's diet can harm both the quality and quantity of her baby's growth. Proteins are essential for the production of brain cells, and a child's future mental capacity may be influenced by protein in the mother's diet. An adequate prenatal supply of protein is directly related to building strong bones and teeth. Children whose mothers lack good protein nutrition tend to have poorer quality bones and teeth than offspring of mothers whose diets contained enough complete protein.

A daily protein intake of 70-80 grams of protein is recommended for pregnant women by the Food and Nutrition Board of the National Academy of Sciences. Many nutritionists, however, consider these figures to be too low and recommend 90 to 100 grams of protein per day, especially during the last half of pregnancy.

Proteins are made up of substances called amino acids. More than 20 different amino acids have been identified. Your body's cells can manufacture all but eight of these. These eight, called "essential" amino acids, must be supplied by your food. "Complete" proteins are those which contain adequate supplies of these eight essential amino acids. "Incomplete" proteins are those which lack completely or have too little of one or more essential amino acids.

If an incomplete protein is eaten at the same time as a complete one such as macaroni and cheese or cereal and milk, the body can combine amino acids to form additional complete proteins. This is also true when certain combinations of two or more incomplete proteins are eaten together (e.g., baked beans and cornbread, or peanut butter on whole wheat bread). Combinations of incomplete proteins are only useful when one supplies the amino acids missing in the other. You'll be surer of meeting your protein nutrition needs if your diet contains an adequate supply of things you know to be complete proteins.

The following sources each provide approximately 15 grams of complete protein. If you select five to six times daily from this list, you will be quite certain of having an adequate supply of protein in your diet.

	SERVING	PROTEIN (Grams)
COTTAGE CHEESE	1/2 cup	15
EGGS	2 large, 3 medium	15
MEAT, FISH, FOWL	3 oz.	20
NATURAL CHEESE (e.g., cheddar, swiss, muenster, Brie)	2 oz.	15
WHOLE MILK (also skim, buttermilk, or yogurt)	2 cups	15
SOYBEANS	3/4 cup cooked	15
WHEAT GERM	1/3 cup	15

Here are some sources of incomplete proteins. Each of the quantities listed supplies about 15 grams of protein. But remember, in order for your body to get the full benefit of these proteins, they must be taken in combination with those that contain the missing essential amino acids.

BEANS (lentils, chick peas, kidney beans)	1 cup, cooked	15
TOFU (bean curd)	2 cakes	15
PASTA (macaroni, noodles)	3 cups, cooked	15
RICE	3 cups, cooked	15

VITAMINS AND MINERALS

During pregnancy, adequate intake of vitamins is especially important. Although most of your vitamin needs can be met through a well-balanced diet, a prenatal vitamin supplement may be prescribed as well. (See page 46.)

VITAMIN A

Vitamin A is a fat-soluble vitamin, which means that the body requires the presence of dietary fats in order to use this vitamin. You should, however, avoid taking mineral oil, because mineral oil is not absorbed by the body and can bind Vitamin A and the other fat-soluble vitamins (D, E, and K) and carry them off so they can't be used as they pass through your digestive system.

Vitamin A is a fat-soluble vitamin, which means that the body must use it in the presence of fats. However, mineral oil, which is not absorbed by the body, should not be taken. Mineral oil can pick up Vitamin A and the other fat-soluble vitamins (D, E, and K) and carry them off so they can't be used as they pass through your digestive system.

Although orange fruits and vegetables, leafy green vegetables, liver and other organ meats are all sources of Vitamin A, prolonged exposure to air or heat of cooking can destroy much of the vitamin before it reaches the table and you.

Because an excess of vitamin A can be stored in body tissues and may cause harm, you shouldn't self prescribe additional quantities of this vitamin. The prenatal vitamins prescribed by your doctor contain a safe amount of Vitamin A when taken as directed.

VITAMIN D

Your body requires Vitamin D in order to regulate the absorption of calcium. Sources of Vitamin D in the diet include fortified milk, egg yolk, margarine, shrimp, salmon, and tuna. If you spend time in the sunlight, Vitamin D can form on the skin and be absorbed. During pregnancy, the recommended daily amount of Vitamin D is 400 IU. Overdose of Vitamin D is possible and should be avoided because it could harm your baby.

VITAMIN E

Vitamin E is necessary for the body's digestion and use of polyunsaturated fats (vegetable oils). It protects them from being destroyed by oxygen. An adequate supply of Vitamin E is related to normal growth patterns and the body's ability to respond to stress.

Diet sources of Vitamin E include wheat germ, whole grains, corn oil, safflower oil, soybean oil, and margarine. Heat, oxygen, and freezing destroy Vitamin E.

If you are taking a vitamin supplement containing E, it's best to take it with a meal containing fats. Take your iron supplement at a different time — preferably eight hours earlier or later. If taken at the same time of day, certain iron supplements (for example, ferrous sulphate) destroy the effectiveness of Vitamin E.

VITAMIN K

Vitamin K is necessary for blood clotting. The body normally can produce an adequate supply of Vitamin K from foodstuffs in the intestine. Sources of this vitamin in the diet are leafy green vegetables such as kale, spinach, or cabbage, beef, pork, cauliflower, carrots, and tomatoes.

VITAMIN C

Vitamin C in sufficient supply is needed for strong cell walls and blood vessels. This vitamin helps the body to utilize Vitamin A, folic acid, and iron. Tender gums and nosebleeds, both common discomforts of pregnancy, are often controlled by an increase of Vitamin C intake. The need for Vitamin C is further increased by stress, disease, or smoking.

You will find Vitamin C in citrus fruits (grapefruits, oranges, lemons, limes, tangerines), melons (cantaloupe, watermelon), strawberries, tomatoes, potatoes, broccoli, cabbage, and kale. You need a fresh supply of Vitamin C every day, because the body doesn't store this vitamin.

Vitamin C is easily destroyed by heat and contact with the air. It dissolves in liquid. Because of this, careful preparation of vegetables containing Vitamin C is required. Don't cook them far in advance, use as little water as possible in cooking, and keep the container covered until serving.

During pregnancy you should stick to the medically recommended quantities of Vitamin C even if you comfortably take very large doses at other times. Remember that your baby is very small, and a safe dose for you could be very much more than the baby could handle. The baby whose system must work hard to deal with overdoses of Vitamin C before birth, may have trouble using Vitamin C effectively later.

B VITAMINS

There are nine generally recognized B-complex vitamins. An adequate supply during pregnancy is necessary for proper cell division and fetal growth. B vitamins aid the body in responding to stress. This can be especially important to you during pregnancy. These vitamins will assist you in digesting carbohydrates and protein. Sufficient quantities of the B vitamins are needed to help prevent certain kinds of anemia.

Toxemia of pregnancy in many cases seems to be related to protein deficient diets. Such cases may be helped by Vitamin B supplements which aid the body in using protein effectively. Severe prenatal deficiencies in Vitamin B_6 have been related to blood disorders and mental retardation. The demand for folic acid appears to increase during pregnancy.

Dietary sources of the B vitamins include whole, unrefined grains (cracked and whole wheat, brown rice, rye, wheat germ), liver and other organ meats, leafy vegetables, milk, and eggs. The B vitamins are quite fragile and are easily destroyed by refining processes or cooking. Because of this, it's often difficult to get enough in your diet. Your doctor may prescribe a supplement.

The B vitamins are water soluble, and excesses are passed out with urine rather than being stored. For this reason, daily intake is necessary. The B vitamins tend to work together, so an individual one should not be omitted or used in significantly larger doses than the others. See the chart on page 33 for the appropriate quantities you need of each of the B vitamins.

IRON

During pregnancy, an increased supply of iron is needed for healthy hemoglobin, the oxygen-carrying substance of your red blood cells. The anemia which results from inadequate iron supply can cause extreme fatigue in the mother as well as reduced oxygen supply to her baby.

Your body will absorb iron more easily if you eat it with foods which are acid (yogurt or those with a high level of Vitamin C). Note that dried apricots, dried prunes, and prune juice can relieve constipation as well as provide iron.

Sources of iron in the diet include:

liver	3 oz.	7-12 mg. of iron
kidney	3 oz.	11 mg.
veal or beef	3 oz.	2-3 mg.
lamb or poultry	3 oz.	2 mg.
wheat germ	1/2 cup	5 mg.
soybeans	1 cup	5 mg.
dried apricots	1/2 cup	4 mg.
dried prunes	4 oz.	3.8 mg.
prune juice	1 cup	10 mg.

Many doctors prescribe an iron supplement, particularly in late pregnancy. If you are taking extra iron, be sure to take it as directed so that your body can benefit from it. Take your iron supplement with a meal, and at a different time of day from your prenatal vitamins.

CALCIUM

A good supply of calcium is important for the development of bones and teeth. If your diet doesn't contain enough calcium, your baby will try to take what it needs from the stored supply in your bones.

If you don't have adequate calcium in your daily diet, you may be irritable and have trouble sleeping. Painful muscle cramps in your legs, as well as pains in the uterus are also thought to be related to calcium deficiency.

Try to get the recommended amount of 1200-1300 mg. of calcium per day. In order to absorb calcium efficiently, your body requires the presence of small to moderate amounts of dietary fat. Whole milk is an efficient source of calcium. Skim milk is also an efficient source, especially if it is consumed at the same time as another source of fat such as lightly buttered toast. Do not, however, use the need to aid calcium absorption as an excuse to consume quantities of fatty foods. Excessive dietary fat can interfere with calcium absorption, and most people get more than enough fat in the diet.

Calcium can combine with substances in certain other foods and take forms that are less easily absorbed. Among these foods which can make the body's use of calcium less efficient are spinach, beet greens, chocolate, candy, or other very concentrated carbohydrates. For example, a glass of chocolate milk will provide less readily usable calcium than a glass of plain milk.

The following foods are good sources of calcium. Each of the quantities listed contains approximately 300 mg. of calcium, the same amount as a half a pint of milk.

cottage cheese	12 oz.
unprocessed cheese	1-1/3 oz.
dry milk powder	1/3 cup
ice cream	1-1/2 cups
yogurt	1 cup
tofu (bean curd)	2 cakes
salmon (canned with bones)	1/2-2/3 cup (depends on brand)

Adding dry powdered milk to hamburger, cereals, baked goods or blender concoctions will increase your intake of calcium. You needn't drink a quart of milk daily in its plain form, as long as you make sure that your daily intake of calcium is adequate. Milk in soups, sauces, puddings, and custards may be more enjoyable. However, be careful not to prepare these items with ingredients which add lots of calories.

Do not use bone meal or dolomite or any preparations containing them as calcium supplements while you are pregnant or nursing your baby. Samples of these mineral supplements have been found to contain dangerously high lead content which could cause serious harm to an unborn child or infant. Lead can cross the placenta and reach the fetus from the mother's body, and it can be transmitted to an infant through the mother's milk.

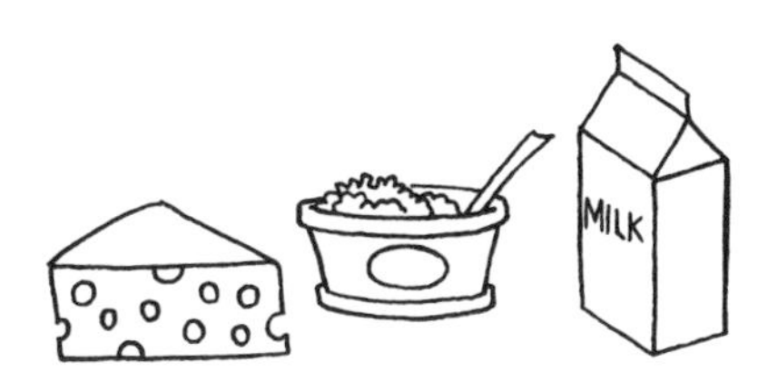

SODIUM

The need to restrict salt in a pregnant woman's diet depends on the individual. During pregnancy, your body may need more sodium than usual because of the increased volume of your circulation. However, many people regularly consume far more salt than they need. If you are one of these people, a restriction in salt intake may be required for you during pregnancy.

If you have a problem with swelling of the legs, hands, or feet, your doctor may advise a salt-restricted diet. If so, try other flavorings such as lemon juice or herbs in your cooking. Read labels carefully. Most canned or packaged foods contain salt. Watch the ingredients listing for any items containing the word sodium, (monosodium glutamate, sodium benzoate, sodium proprionate, etc.).

SODIUM RESTRICTED DIETS

Sodium is a mineral which is found in some quantity in nearly every food. Because most of what you eat naturally contains some sodium, it is easy to meet the body's daily requirement for this mineral without adding extra salt (which is 40% sodium) to anything you prepare. Sources of sodium in addition to table salt are monosodium glutamate (MSG), baking soda and baking powder, and a number of preservatives and other materials used in food processing.

It may be advisable for some pregnant women to limit their intake of sodium. Here are some guidelines to help you plan your meals if your doctor suggests a sodium restricted diet for you.

- Don't add salt when you cook. Keep the salt shaker off the table.
- Avoid salted snack foods such as potato chips, crackers, crisps, pretzels, or salted peanuts. Stay away from olives or pickles.
- Fresh vegetables are fine. Canned or frozen vegetables should be avoided unless they have been processed without salt. Commercially processed cans and packages of vegetables contain salt unless the label specifically tells you otherwise.
- Avoid maraschino cherries and fruits preserved with benzoate of soda. Fresh fruits are fine. Canned and frozen fruits are generally O.K. but are often a source of unneeded sugar. Make sure the jams, jellies, and marmalade you use do not contain sodium benzoate.
- Stay away from all salted, canned, or smoked meats and fish. Avoid frozen fish fillets. Shellfish (other than oysters) are high in sodium and should be avoided. Stick with fresh meat and fish prepared without salt.
- Fast food places generally use salt in preparation. Avoid their burgers, fish fillets, or other entrees. Stay away from hot dogs and cold cuts.
- Use unsalted butter and unsalted cottage cheese. Avoid all other cheeses.
- Use homemade soups made without salt. Don't use bullion cubes, canned soups, or instant soup packages.
- Avoid desserts prepared with salt, baking powder or soda, or egg whites. Packaged gelatin desserts, puddings, and many commercially packaged ice creams should also be avoided. Read the labels.
- Avoid ordinary bread, quick breads, rolls, and ready-to-bake packaged items. Stay away from crackers and soda crackers.

- Cooked cereal prepared without salt is all right. Don't use the instant packages or quick-cooking variety. Most commercially packed dry cereals contain too much sodium and should be avoided.
- Avoid seasonings and condiments that contain sodium. The obvious ones are items such as garlic salt, onion salt, or celery salt. For many others, however, you'll have to read the ingredients as well as the name on the label. (One brand of "lemon and pepper seasoning," for example, contains salt as its major ingredient.) Stay away from catsup, mustard, Worcestershire sauce, steak sauce, soy sauce, and horseradish prepared with salt.
- Don't use meat tenderizers.
- Avoid commercially prepared salad dressings. Make your own with unsalted oil and vinegar. Try seasonings such as pepper, lemon juice, garlic, oregano, poultry seasoning, sage, or thyme.
- Most diet sodas contain more sodium than their regular counterparts. It's generally best to avoid all carbonated beverages.

Read the labels carefully when you buy. Ingredients are listed in descending order by quantity. The closer salt is to the beginning of the list, the more there is relative to the other ingredients. Avoid foods with a listed ingredient of salt or any other containing the word sodium.

If you dine out, you should go to restaurants where the food is prepared to order so that your meal can be prepared without salt. Avoid Chinese restaurants which use MSG in the preparation of many dishes unless you are sure dishes can be prepared to meet your special needs.

FLUIDS

You should drink at least two quarts or more (8-10 glasses) of liquid a day while you're pregnant. Good sources of fluid in addition to water are unsweetened fruit and vegetable juices. Avoid drinks which have a lot of sugar added, such as fruit punches or ades, because they provide unnecessary calories.

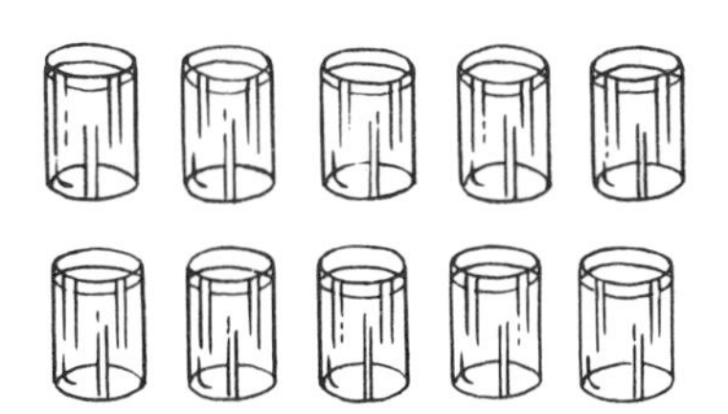

Carbonated beverages should be avoided because they have little or no nutritional value and they produce gas which may make you uncomfortable. Regular sodas are very high in calories. Diet sodas, on the other hand, contain potentially dangerous additives such as saccharin or aspartame, and they often have more than double the sodium content of regular sodas. You'll be better off if you stick to clear beverages.

Another disadvantage of carbonated beverages is that the bubbles increase the surface area of food available for exposure to digestive enzymes, thus enabling the enzymes to act more rapidly and completely. While this may cause you to derive more energy from certain foods, it will also increase the caloric intake.

FOOD ADDITIVES

Additives of one sort or another are included in most processed foods today. Some are safe, and some are not. A number of them have not been tested thoroughly enough to be sure. During pregnancy, it's best to be very careful and plan your meals so that additives which might be dangerous are avoided whenever possible. This chart will help you do that.

DROP THESE FROM YOUR DIET

WHAT	FOUND IN	WHY
Food Colorings (especially Orange B, Red No. 3, Red No. 40, Yellow No. 5, Blue No. 1 and Blue No. 2)	Artificial coloring is found in a wide variety of products from hot dogs to candy.	Most are poorly tested. Some are known to cause cancer in laboratory animals. Some are suspected of causing hyperactivity. All are unnecessary.
Artificial Flavorings	Hundreds of different chemicals are used instead of natural flavors. They are identified only as "artificial flavor" on the label.	These are often found in junk foods. The real thing may be more nutritious. Some may cause hyperactivity. Foods containing artificial flavoring are not needed in your diet.
BHT (Butylated Hydroxytoluene)	This antioxidant is used as a preservative in cereals, potato chips, oils, chewing gum, etc.	When stored in the body, may cause allergic reactions, possibly cancer. BHT is banned in Great Britain from foods intended for children.
BHA (Butylated Hydroxyanisole)	This antioxidant is used as a preservative in oils, cereals, potato chips, chewing gum, etc.	This seems to be somewhat safer than BHT, but no one knows for sure. Like BHT, it is banned in Great Britain.
MSG (Monosodium Glutamate)	This is a flavor enhancer used in soups, poultry, seafood, stews, sauces, Chinese cooking, and many packaged convenience foods and specialty items.	MSG is known to injure brain cells of baby mice in lab experiments. It can cause headaches and "Chinese restaurant syndrome," a burning feeling and tightness in the face, head, neck, and arms.
Caffein	This stimulant is found naturally in tea, coffee, and cocoa. It is added to cola drinks.	Too much caffeine may cause you trouble in getting to sleep. Heavy use may be related to birth defects or miscarriage.
Quinine	This is a flavoring used in tonic or quinine water, or bitter lemon.	Quinine is not well tested. It may cause birth defects.
Saccharin Aspartame	These are both artificial sweeteners used in diet sodas and foods.	Saccharin is known to cause cancer in laboratory animals. Aspartame is suspected of causing brain damage in sensitive individuals. A fetus may be at risk for these effects.
Sodium Nitrite and Sodium Nitrate	These are used to preserve, color, and flavor bacon, ham, hot dogs, corned beef, lunch meats, etc.	Especially in fried bacon, these can cause formation of small quantities of nitrosamines which can cause cancer.

BE CAREFUL WITH THESE

WHAT	FOUND IN	WHY
Phosphoric Acid Phosphates	These are used in baked goods, cured meats, cereals, dried potatoes, soda.	Although they are not toxic, their wide use may lead to dietary imbalance that might cause osteoporosis.
Propyl Gallate	This antioxidant is used in meat products, potato sticks, some chicken soup, chewing gum.	This is not well tested. Although no serious dangers are suspected, it's often unnecessary.
Sulfur Dioxide Sodium Bisulfate	These preservative and bleaching agents are found in sliced fruit, wine, grape juice, dried potatoes, and dried fruit.	These are safe, but they can destroy Vitamin B_1.

The additives listed above are the ones you should watch for most carefully. Many additives are safe and necessary. When you read a label, don't be fooled by long names that are hard to read. Current government regulations require that many ingredients be listed by their technical chemical name. Some of these are things that have been known by other names and used safely for years.

The source for information in this chart is "Chemical Cuisine," a poster from the Center for Science in the Public Interest, Washington, D.C.

FATS

Fats are found in animal protein foods such as milk, meat, and egg yolks. Other important sources in the diet are grains, nuts, seeds, and the oils made from them. Among the nutrients supplied by fats in your diet is linoleic acid, an essential fatty acid which your body can't manufacture on its own. Fats provide energy, and aid in the absorption of calcium and Vitamin A. If your diet contains the suggested animal proteins and grain products, it is likely to contain sufficient amounts of fats.

VEGETARIAN DIETS

It is possible to meet the nutrition requirements on a vegetarian diet during pregnancy, although this is very difficult. A pregnant vegetarian must have and use detailed knowledge of the nutritional values of everything she will eat. She must know which incomplete proteins complement each other to form complete proteins. She must be sure to eat these protein foods in proper quantity and combination.

If you are a vegetarian and intend to continue to be during your pregnancy, discuss this with your doctor. To give your baby the best possible start in life, you may wish to consider adding certain items (such as fish or poultry) to your diet until after your baby is born.

PRENATAL VITAMINS

Many doctors feel that prenatal vitamins are added insurance that you and your baby are getting all the vitamins you need. It is true that most vitamin needs could be met through a well balanced diet. However, it's often difficult to tell for sure what you are getting from your food alone. Many vitamins can be destroyed or weakened during food processing or preparation. A vitamin supplement is an extra safeguard.

If you are taking vitamin supplements prescribed by your doctor, keep in mind that they are not a substitute for eating well. You can't swallow the pill and skip the meal.

VITAMINS IN MASSIVE DOSES

Some people today take massive doses of certain vitamins because they believe there are certain health or nutrition values to doing this. No matter what your personal views might be about large doses of vitamins, pregnancy is a time to avoid this practice. While your body may be able to cope comfortably with large amounts of vitamins, this same quantity could damage your baby. Remember that your unborn child is very small, and what's comfortable for you could be a harmful overdose for your baby.

NUTRITION FOR PREGNANT TEENAGERS

During pregnancy, your body has increased nutritional needs of its own in addition to the nutritional requirements of your developing baby. It is essential to eat properly during pregnancy regardless of your pre-pregnancy weight. Pregnancy is neither a time to diet for weight loss, nor a time to indulge in quantities of foods that are fattening but not nutritious.

For a typical mother who eats wisely during pregnancy, here's what the recommended 24 pound gain might include.

WEIGHT GAIN

No matter what your weight was before you became pregnant, you must eat properly now to support your own body's increased needs and the needs of your developing baby. While pregnancy is not a time to diet for weight loss, neither is it a time to indulge in quantities of foods that are fattening but not nutritious.

For a typical mother who eats wisely during pregnancy, here's what the recommended 24 pound gain might include.

BABY	7-1/2 pounds	BLOOD	3-1/2 pounds
PLACENTA	1-1/2 pounds	OTHER FLUID	2-3/4 pounds
AMNIOTIC FLUID	2 pounds	UTERUS	2-1/2 pounds
BREAST TISSUE	1 pound	OTHER	3-1/4 pounds

Section Four

FOR YOUR INFORMATION

Acne and Accutane / Addictive Drugs / AIDS / Alcohol / Alpha Fetoprotein Tests / Alternative Birth Settings / Amniocentesis / Amniotomy / Aspartame / Automobile Safety / Baths / Breech Presentation / Caesarean Delivery / Caffeine / Chorionic Villi Sampling (CVS) / Dental Work / Diabetes / Dilation and Effacement / Disability Benefits / Diuretics / Douching / Ectopic Pregnancy / Electronic Fetal Monitoring / Employment / Enema / Episiotomy / Estriol Tests / Exercise / Induced Labor / Leboyer Delivery / Lovemaking / Marijuana / Medications (during pregnancy) / Medications (for labor and delivery) / Miscarriage / Nipple Care / Nonstress Test / Oxytocin Challenge Test (Stress Test) / Pregnancy Loss / Prep / Prepared Childbirth / Rh-Negative Mothers / Rooming-In / Rubella / Saunas and Hot Tubs / Sibling Participation / Smoking / Sports / Tampons / Toxemia of Pregnancy / Toxic Substances / Toxoplasmosis / Travel / Twins / Ultrasound / VBAC (Vaginal Birth After Caesarean) / Venereal Disease / Weight / X-rays

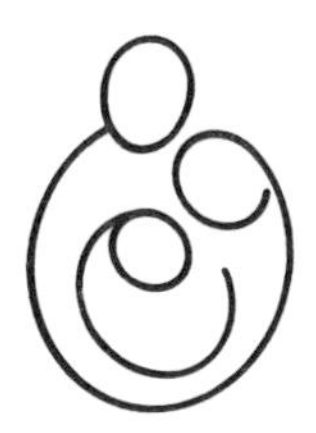

FOR YOUR INFORMATION

The following section of WHILE WAITING contains an alphabetical listing of topics about which many women have questions. Here you will find guidelines for activities and personal health care during your pregnancy. Brief explanations of certain medical procedures and terms can also be found in this section. If you have further questions about any of the listed items, or questions about things not included here, BE SURE TO ASK.

You or your doctor should note here any topics that are especially important reading for your particular situation.

______________________	page ___	______________________	page ___
______________________	page ___	______________________	page ___
______________________	page ___	______________________	page ___

ACNE AND ACCUTANE

Accutane is a prescription medication used in the treatment of severe cystic acne. Accutane, first marketed in late 1982, is very effective in relieving facial acne scars, but it is also known to cause serious birth defects if used by a pregnant woman. Among the problems associated with Accutane use during pregnancy are babies born with abnormalities of the brain, ears, face, and thymus gland, along with some degree of mental retardation.

A pregnancy test to make sure you are not pregnant is advised before beginning a course of acne treatment using Accutane. If you know you are pregnant, or plan to become pregnant within the near future, do not use Accutane even if it has been prescribed for you in the past by a dermatologist or other physician.

ADDICTIVE DRUGS

We do know that the placenta does not protect the fetus from the mother's use of drugs such as cocaine, heroin, or LSD. It is not just illegal drugs that may cause harm. An addictive substance such as valium, even if it was prescribed for you under other circumstances, should not be taken during pregnancy. Use of such drugs during pregnancy has been associated with various birth defects including brain damage and physical abnormalities.

If a woman uses addictive drugs in moderate to heavy doses it is likely that her baby will go through a very painful period of withdrawal right after birth. The use of such drugs, especially during pregnancy, is not recommended.

AIDS

AIDS (acquired immune deficiency syndrome) is a viral disease that destroys the immune system of its victims. AIDS is most prevalent among male homosexuals and intravenous drug users, although it is not confined to these groups. AIDS is not thought to be contagious through casual contact. However, if either parent has AIDS or is a carrier of the disease, a child born to these parents may be at risk of developing AIDS. There is some evidence that the second pregnancy of a woman carrying the AIDS virus or diagnosed as having AIDS may be more dangerous than the first pregnancy—for mother and for the baby.

There is much about AIDS that we don't know at this time. If you suspect that the disease may be a problem for you or your partner, consult your physician for further information.

ALCOHOL

If you drink, you should keep in mind that the placenta does not keep alcohol away from your unborn child. Every time you take a drink, so does your baby. It takes the baby about one hour to get free from the immediate effects of a single ounce of alcohol.

Although some research has suggested that the effects of alcohol on a developing baby are only temporary, we are now learning that this may not always be so. Heavy drinking replaces the intake of nutritious foods, and this too may cause harm.

The U.S. Surgeon General's office advises that pregnant women drink no alcohol.

Children of heavy drinkers may be born with Fetal Alcohol Syndrome (FAS), the name now given to an identifiable pattern of physical and mental difficulties. These babies may be smaller and less well formed, with physical problems such as kidney disorders, heart defects, or facial abnormalities. Some FAS babies are mentally retarded. Less severely affected infants may have lower birth weight, learning disabilities, and a tendency to be hyperactive or irritable.

We do not know how much drinking is too much, but we do know that it is not just the daily drinker who is at risk. An occasional crash binge with great amounts of wine, beer, or liquor consumed at one time may also cause harm. It's best to save any celebrations involving alcohol until after your baby is born.

If you would like to stop drinking and are having trouble, feel free to talk about it during a visit to your doctor. Your medical team is there to help.

ALPHA FETOPROTEIN TESTS

A measure of alpha fetoprotein may be used for prenatal detection of neural tube defects (birth defects such as spinabifida or anencephaly). This screening is usually done by means of a blood test between 15 and 20 weeks of pregnancy. If the blood test shows an elevated AFP level, a repeat of the test may be suggested. If necessary, additional diagnostic procedures such as ultrasound (see page 69) or amniocentesis (see page 50) will be used to evaluate the possibility of neural tube defects. If, because of other risk factors such as age or family history, a woman has already elected to have amniocentesis, the alpha fetoprotein level can be tested in the amniotic fluid. In such cases, the blood screening test for AFP level would not be an additional requirement.

ALTERNATIVE BIRTH SETTINGS

To achieve a family-centered birthing experience in a homelike setting, but without the potential hazards of home birth, many women are turning to alternative birth settings either within a hospital or affiliated with one.

In direct response to consumer demand, many hospitals now offer birthing rooms in which a woman may labor, deliver, recover, and enjoy bonding with her newborn all in the same place before moving to the regular maternity/nursery facilities. In some hospitals, birthing room facilities may be limited, and available on a first come, first served basis. If such is the case, making your request known early may be helpful.

A number of hospitals have taken the birthing room concept one step further and have established alternative birth centers separate from the regular obstetric units. These alternative centers, which offer maximum homelike flexibility and minimum intervention, are often limited to those women classified as "low risk."

Another option for low-risk women is a birth center outside the hospital. In these centers most deliveries are handled by nurse-midwives, and the emphasis is on viewing birth as a normal process. These birth centers have backup arrangements with nearby hospitals in case additional medical intervention is required.

AMNIOCENTESIS

Amniocentesis is a diagnostic procedure in which a needle is inserted into the womb of a pregnant woman and a small amount of amniotic fluid is removed. Laboratory examination (a process which takes 3-4 weeks) of the fluid's cells can detect the presence of a number of genetic defects, and also identify the sex of the fetus.

Perhaps the most common use of amniocentesis is among women over 35 to detect the presence of Down's syndrome, a chromosome abnormality which results in a child with mental retardation and physical malformation. The chances of bearing a child with Down's syndrome increase sharply with age. Amniocentesis can also detect diseases such as sickle cell anemia (common among blacks) and Tay-Sachs disease (found among Eastern European Jews).

Amniocentesis to detect genetic defects is usually done during the 13th to 16th week of pregnancy. A woman might choose to terminate a pregnancy if she finds that she is carrying a child with a particular genetic disorder. For a woman at risk to find out that her child does not have the feared genetic defect would be reassuring. Ruling out these disorders does not, however, guarantee a healthy baby. There are many birth defects which can not be determined by amniocentesis.

Amniocentesis may also be used later in pregnancy to assess the health and development of the fetus. For example, analysis of the amniotic fluid can determine the degree of fetal lung maturity. This information could be of vital importance in medical decision making should there be reasons to contemplate delivery before term.

Amniocentesis is expensive and it is not completely without risk to the fetus. However, in cases of advanced maternal age or certain family backgrounds, the benefits of the information obtained may outweigh the risks of the procedure. If you have questions about amniocentesis, you should discuss the pros and cons of it with your doctor to decide if it is an appropriate procedure for you.

AMNIOTOMY

Amniotomy is the intentional rupture of the membranes (breaking of the bag of waters) surrounding the baby. This procedure, done with a sterile instrument, causes no pain for the mother. Amniotomy is used to induce or speed up labor, and to permit the insertion of an internal electronic fetal monitor.

Amniotomy is a vey commonly used intervention. Those opposed to its use point out that the amniotic sac does offer some protection to the baby's head during labor. It is possible for a baby to be born with the bag of waters still intact. If you have any questions about the use of this procedure in your case, ask your doctor or midwife.

ASPARTAME

Aspartame, approved in 1981 for sale in the United States, is a widely used artificial sweetener. Aspartame is marketed as a sugar sweetener under the trade name Equal. As the food additive NutraSweet, it is found in a variety of products from diet sodas to breakfast foods and packaged desserts.

Although aspartame is popular and generally regarded as safe, some researchers have suggested that high doses of aspartame may be associated with problems ranging from dizziness and subtle brain changes to mental retardation. The effects of aspartame vary with individual sensitivity to the substance. Pregnant women and their babies may be more susceptible to the effects of aspartame than a non-pregnant adult would be.

During pregnancy, you should not use products containing aspartame. The amount of the sweetener, if any, that might be a safe dose for an unborn child is not known at this time.

AUTOMOBILE SAFETY

Being pregnant is not a reason to stop driving your car, so long as you feel up to it and fit behind the wheel while still reaching the pedals. Whether you are the driver or a passenger, you should be careful not to sit for extended periods of time. Stop the car every hour or so and walk around for a few minutes to stimulate your circulation.

When you are pregnant, just as when you are not, wearing a safety belt greatly increases your chances of avoiding serious injury or death in an automobile accident. A pregnant woman should fasten the safety belt so the lap part of the belt is snugly across her upper thighs and under her protruding abodomen. The shoulder part of the restraint must also be used for the device to function properly. The shoulder strap is best positioned between the breasts, if possible.

If you are tempted to use your pregnancy as an excuse not to bother with seat belts, here are some facts you should consider:

- The commonly held belief that seat belts may harm an unborn child is a myth that has no basis in fact. A correctly positioned seat belt does not increase the chances of fetal injury in a survivable collision.
- Don't be concerned that the safety belt shoulder strap will harm your breasts. Even in a collision which temporarily causes a breast to be pressed by the strap, no serious damage to the breast is likely.
- Most automobile accidents occur within 25 miles of home. You and your unborn child need the protection of a safety restraint system even on those short trips to the shopping mall or your doctor's office.
- A major cause of death of an unborn child in an automobile accident is death of the mother. Using a safety restraint system can save your life, and your baby's life along with it.

Before your baby is born, you should obtain an infant restraint system if you plan to transport your baby by car. Beginning with the trip home from the hospital, be sure to secure your child in an approved safety seat **every time** you travel by automobile.

BATHS

You may take tub baths or showers, whichever you prefer, throughout your pregnancy. The temperature of your bath water should not exceed 100 degrees, as extremely hot water could harm your developing baby. This is especially true during the first three months. You should avoid saunas and health club hot tubs as well as overheated home baths during pregnancy. As your size and weight increase, be careful not to lose your balance getting in and out of the bathtub.

If your bag of waters has broken, do not take a tub bath. There is a danger of infection once the membranes have ruptured. Take a shower instead.

Important

During pregnancy, your bath water should be 100° or less. Extremely hot temperatures can cause fetal damage.

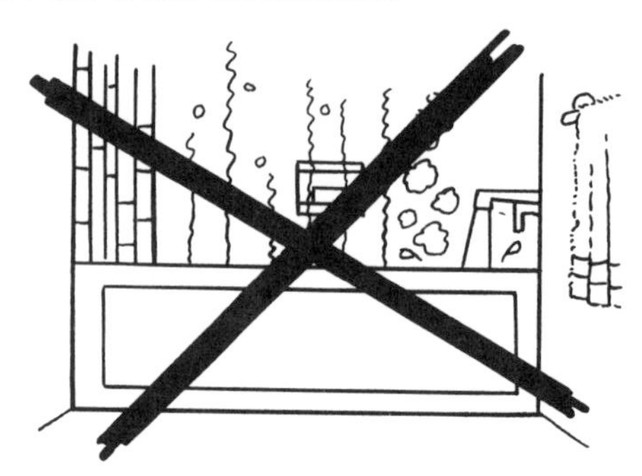

BREECH PRESENTATION

More than 95% of the babies delivered present themselves in a head first position. Occasionally, however, the baby is turned so that the buttocks or another body part is closest to the cervix. This is called a breech presentation. Sometimes a baby in a breech position will turn naturally before labor. Sometimes the doctor will be able to turn the baby. Although it is possible for a baby to be born other than head first, many breech presentations require a Caesarean section. Your doctor will discuss this with you if necessary.

CAESAREAN DELIVERY

You should keep in mind that a Caesarean delivery is always a possibility, although for many women that possibility is a small one. In some situations — for example, small pelvic opening and large baby, or certain breech presentations — the need for a Caesarean can be predicted in advance and you will have a chance to prepare for it. In other cases — for example, fetal distress — the decision for a Caesarean will be made on the spot by the doctor during your labor.

In a Caesarean delivery, the doctor makes a surgical incision in your abdomen and uterus and removes the baby. Before a Caesarean is done, you will be asked to sign permission for the operation. A small amount of blood will be drawn for analysis. To prepare your body for the operation, your abdomen will be shaved and you will receive an I-V and a urinary catheter.

Caesarean deliveries generally work out well for both mother and baby, although the recovery time may be slightly longer for the mother than it would be for a vaginal delivery. In many hospitals, your partner may stay with you for the birth if the two of you and your doctor are comfortable with the idea. You can breastfeed your baby if you wish, although for the first day or two you may need help placing the baby in a comfortable position for you.

If you have any questions about the possible need for a Caesarean in your case, please ask. If a Caesarean is required, feel free to ask about any of the procedures as they occur.

It was once thought that a woman who delivered one baby by Caesarean section would be required to have any future children by this means as well. This is no longer correct. Depending on the reason for the first Caesarean and your present condition, delivery of your baby vaginally may be not only possible but also preferable to another Caesarean. Discuss this with your doctor well in advance of your due date. (See VBAC, Vaginal Birth After Caesarean, page 69.)

CAFFEINE

Recent studies suggest a relationship between excessive consumption of caffeine during pregnancy and birth defects. Although moderate amounts may not be harmful, it's best to limit your intake of coffee, tea, cola beverages, or other items containing caffeine. Caffeine is a stimulant and it does cross the placenta to your baby. If you feel the need for a cup of coffee to get going in the morning, that's probably all right. However, frequent coffee breaks during the day could cause trouble. Furthermore, the person who drinks too much coffee, tea, or cola may tend to neglect other beverages with greater nutritional value.

CHORIONIC VILLI SAMPLING (CVS)

Chorionic villi sampling is a procedure that analyzes samples of placental tissue to assess fetal wellbeing. Some medical centers now offer CVS as an alternative to amniocentesis. The technique can be used at 10 to 12 weeks of pregnancy, and the results obtained about two weeks after that. In a case where pregnancy termination is an option the woman would consider, the early availability of information is an advantage. Disadvantages include a somewhat higher rate of failure to obtain information, and a slightly higher rate of spontaneous abortion (miscarriage) following the procedure.

DENTAL WORK

Your mouth's normal bacteria and acid/alkaline balance change during pregnancy, and this may make you more prone to cavities at this time. It's good to visit your dentist early in your pregnancy and have a thorough professional cleaning of your teeth and gums. This may help prevent the tenderness and inflammation of gums that many women experience during pregnancy.

Be sure to inform your dentist that you are pregnant. X-rays should be avoided during the first four months. If absolutely necessary later in your pregnancy, dental X-rays may be done using a protective shield. However, it's better to wait until after your baby is born if you can do so.

DIABETES

Diabetes is a disease in which there is an imbalance between sugar in the body and the body's insulin supply. This imbalance and its effects may intensify during pregnancy, with serious consequences for both mother and fetus. Before the availability of synthetic insulin, the pregnancy of a diabetic woman had little chance for a successful outcome. Now, however, careful medical monitoring can help a diabetic woman increase her chances of having a healthy baby.

A diabetic pregnancy is a high risk one. If you are diabetic, it's especially important that you follow recommendations regarding diet and medication, and that you see your physician for regular checkups. Your appointments will be scheduled on a more frequent basis than they would be for most pregnant women. Diabetics are more likely to develop toxemia, have stillbirths during the last two weeks or so of term, or have abnormally large babies. For these reasons, delivery by Caesarean section before term is sometimes indicated.

A small number of women develop diabetes during pregnancy even though they have no previous history of the disease. If you should develop gestational diabetes, as this condition is called, you will be carefully monitored for the rest of your pregnancy. Excessive weight gain may be a warning sign for cases of gestational diabetes.

DILATION AND EFFACEMENT

Before your baby can enter the birth canal, the mouth of your uterus (cervix) must thin out (efface) and open (dilate). This process of effacement and dilation may begin before you actually go into labor. At each of your office visits during the last month of pregnancy, the doctor may do an internal examination to check on the effacement and dilation of your cervix. The amount of effacement is reported in percent. For example, a cervix which is thinned out three fourths of the way is said to be 75% effaced. Dilation is measured in centimeters or fingers. One finger equals approximately two centimeters.

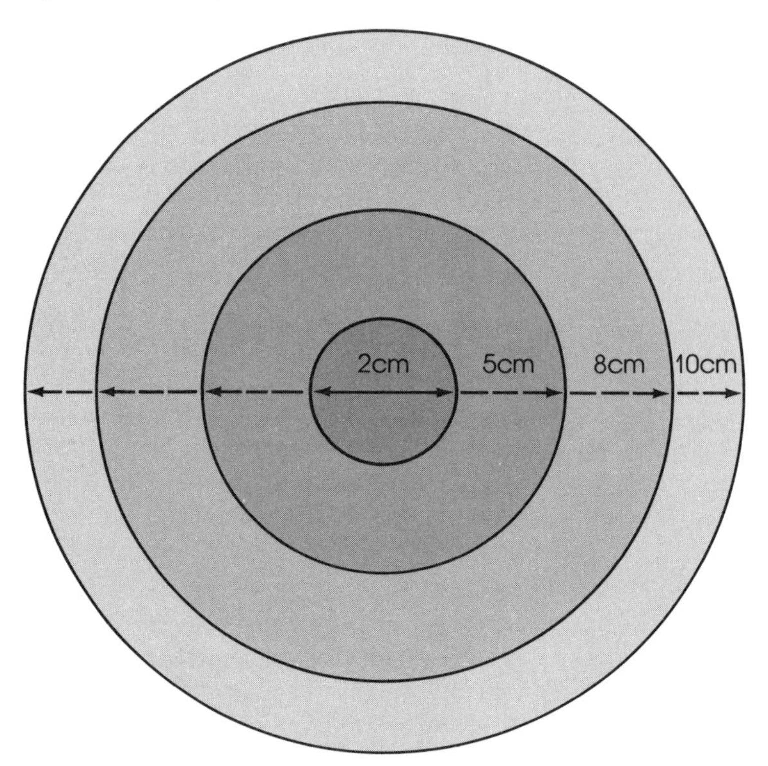

During the first stage of labor (see pages 84 to 87), the cervix effaces fully and dilates to about ten centimeters (five fingers) so that the baby's head can get through. The first stage of labor ends when the cervix is fully effaced and dilated. The following illustrations, from left to right, will give you an idea of how the cervix effaces and dilates during the first stage of labor.

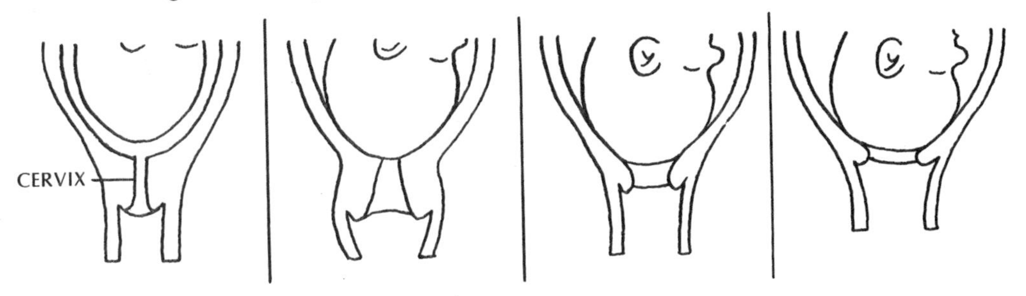

DISABILITY BENEFITS

If you are employed during your pregnancy, you may be entitled to certain sick leave and/or disability benefits from your employer. Although pregnancy is not an illness, the law requires that it be treated in the same way as other temporary disabilities for purposes of sick leave or disability insurance. So, if you are unable to work because of your pregnancy, you should check with your employer to see what benefits, if any, are provided.

DIURETICS

In the past, diuretics (water pills) were routinely prescribed to help a pregnant woman reduce the swelling in the legs caused by fluid retention. They are no longer used freely. This type of medication flushes out needed substances along with the unwanted fluids, and continued use may harm the baby. (See page 23 for alternative ways of dealing with the problem of fluid retention.)

Never take a diuretic on your own when you are pregnant. Although these medications should not be used routinely in pregnancy, one might be prescribed when dietary and other measures have failed and the medical risks of letting the condition continue are greater than the risks of the medication. If your doctor prescribes a diuretic for you at any time, be sure to ask any questions you might have.

DOUCHING

Unless your doctor orders it and explains how to go about it, do not douche during pregnancy. Unlike any other time, it is now possible to introduce air into your circulatory system under pressure from the douche solution. This can cause serious complications, even death. Also, late in your pregnancy, you could break your bag of waters.

ECTOPIC PREGNANCY

In a routine pregnancy, the fertilized ovum moves down the fallopian tube into the uterus where it implants and develops. However, in a very small percentage of cases something goes wrong and the pregnancy develops in the tube or, in extremely rare instances, in the abdominal or pelvic area outside the womb. This is called an ectopic (meaning "out-of-place") pregnancy. Failure to identify and remove an ectopic pregnancy can result in hemorrhage and even death for the mother.

Signs of an ectopic pregnancy may include any or all of the following: sharp or dull pain, erratic vaginal bleeding, weakness or dizziness, headaches, and pain in the neck or shoulder (caused by excessive blood in the pelvis). If you experience any of these symptoms, consult your doctor without delay.

ELECTRONIC FETAL MONITORING

Electronic fetal monitoring is a means of continuously observing the baby's heartbeat to check his or her condition in the womb during labor. There are two types of electronic monitoring: internal and external. The internal monitor uses an electrode attached to the baby's scalp to record fetal heart rate. An electrode placed inside the mother's uterus records contractions. An internal fetal monitor can't be used until the membranes have ruptured spontaneously or an amniotomy has been performed. The external monitor, which is less accurate than the internal one, is strapped around the mother's abdomen and uses ultrasound to record contractions and fetal heart rate.

The alternative to electronic fetal monitoring is fetal monitoring by a nurse or other birth attendant using a stethoscope. With a one-nurse-per-laboring-woman ratio, monitoring by a trained person has been shown to be as reliable and safe for the baby as monitoring electronically. Some labouring women prefer not to be attached to a device that limits their freedom to move around the room and to assume any position they find comfortable. Others, however, feel more secure when monitored electronically.

Some hospitals and physicians use electronic fetal monitoring routinely in all labors. Others employ the devices only when specifically indicated for high risk deliveries. Routine use of electronic monitoring has been associated with an increase in the chances of Caesarean delivery. If you wish, you may discuss with your doctor in advance whether or not electronic fetal monitoring will be required during your labor. Feel free to ask any questions you may have.

EMPLOYMENT

You may continue working as long as you wish. Years ago, some employers discriminated against women who were pregnant and set arbitrary limits on the length of time a pregnant woman could continue on the job. Such attitudes, however, are no longer legally permitted or medically recommended. Many women choose to work throughout their nine months.

If you suspect that the nature of your job may place you or your baby at risk, (e.g., microchip production, exposure to radiation or hazardous chemicals) discuss this with your prenatal caregivers early in your pregnancy. If your job is physically strenuous, talk with your doctor about a comfortable level of physical activity when you approach the beginning of the last trimester (seventh month) of your pregnancy, or sooner if you feel the need. If your job requires you to sit, it's important to get up and walk around for a few minutes every hour or two. This will help prevent circulation slowdown and possible clot formation. (See also DISABILITY BENEFITS, and TOXIC SUBSTANCES.)

ENEMA

In many hospitals, an enema for a laboring woman is a routine procedure following admission. The purpose of the enema is to empty the lower bowel to give the baby more room. For many women, nature provides its own cleansing process and bowel movements or diarrhea empty the bowels naturally before or during early labor. If you have already emptied your bowels naturally, you should be able to choose not to have an enema. Discuss this with your birth attendant.

EPISIOTOMY

An episiotomy is an incision in the perineum (area between the vagina and anus) to enlarge the birth opening. Its purpose is to keep the perineum from tearing and to hasten delivery. If you have an episiotomy, it will be done just before the baby's head is delivered. After the baby is born and the placenta delivered, the incision will be stitched. A local anesthetic such as novocaine will be used before the episiotomy is repaired, unless, of course, you have already had a general or regional anesthetic. (See page 96 for suggestions on how to ease the discomfort from an episiotomy as the incision heals.)

Some doctors do episioitomies routinely. Others evaluate the need for one on a case by case basis. You may wish to discuss with your doctor in advance whether an episiotomy might be likely in your situation.

You can help increase your chance of delivery without an episiotomy or tearing by doing the Kegel exercises described on page 26. These exercises, if done regularly, will prepare and strengthen your perineum for delivery.

ESTRIOL TESTS

Estriol is an estrogen produced by the fetal-placental unit in increasing amounts as pregnancy progresses. Estriol is excreted in the mother's urine, where it can be measured if necessary. Testing the level of estriol in the urine and blood can provide important information about how well the placenta is functioning. Estriol tests may be ordered for a mother with diabetes, toxemia, or severe hypertension, or if a baby is thought to be too small or considerably overdue. A significant drop in estriol level from one test to another may indicate the need to induce labor.

For an estriol test, you must collect in one container all your urine for 24 hours. Your doctor's office or laboratory will supply the container and instructions for when to begin and where to bring the completed sample. You should refrigerate the urine you've collected. You must include every bit of urine for the 24 hours. Be careful, lest you forget and flush away part of the sample.

An alternative to testing estriol in the urine is analysis of the estriol level in the mother's blood. The necessary blood sample can be drawn in your doctor's office. This test provides the same information for making decisions that the urine estriol test does.

EXERCISE

Without a doubt, a regular program of exercise enhances your physical condition and comfort not only during pregnancy, but during labor and delivery and afterwards. If your body feels good, you will be happier and more confident.

Swimming or walking will benefit your entire body, and are especially good sources of exercise during pregnancy. A brisk daily walk may help prevent circulatory problems. (See SPORTS for additional information.)

The pelvic floor (Kegel) exercises beginning on page 26, and the exercises for abdominal muscles on page 29 are designed especially to help you strengthen muscles you will use in labor and delivery. You will find these exercises useful after your baby is born as well.

INDUCED LABOR

Labor can be started by the artificial rupture of membranes or by using the synthetic hormone oxytocin, which is given in an I-V. In the past, babies born "by appointment" were not uncommon because some doctors routinely induced labor and mothers often requested it. This practice, however, is now known to contain potential hazards for both mother and baby, and is not generally recommended.

There are certain medical reasons to induce labor. These reasons include illness of the mother such as toxemia or diabetes, or deterioration of placental functioning. In these cases, onset of labor is necessary for the health of the mother, the baby, or both. Convenience — yours or your doctor's — is not a medical reason for induction. So, even if you feel sure you have been pregnant too long, in most cases it's best to let nature take its course. If an induced labor is suggested for you, feel free to ask about the reasons.

LEBOYER DELIVERY

This approach to delivery, developed by the French obstetrician Frederick Leboyer, is an effort to minimize trauma to the newborn by providing a gentle, loving atmosphere for birth. Leboyer's recommendations include a quiet and dimly lit environment, the immediate placement of the newborn on the mother's abdomen, waiting to cut the cord until it has stopped pulsating, and giving the baby a warm bath to ease the transition from the womb to the outside world. If this approach to delivery interests you, try reading Birth Without Violence, by Frederick Leboyer, M.D. It was published in 1975 by Alfred A. Knopf, New York.

LOVEMAKING

Unless there is a specific problem with your pregnancy which your doctor will discuss with you, you may make love throughout your nine months. No harm will come to you or your baby.

Oral sex during pregnancy is permissible if you enjoy it, but we caution you and your partner not to allow air to be blown into your vagina. Because of the way your body's circulatory system has changed to accommodate your pregnancy, it is possible for air bubbles (emboli) to enter your bloodstream at this time and cause serious damage, even death.

For some people sexual desire is enhanced during pregnancy, for others it is lessened. As your shape changes, you may be more comfortable with different positions or methods. Talking together about your feelings at this time will help you to understand yourself and each other.

MARIJUANA

Most of the reasons not to smoke cigarettes during pregnancy (see pages 64-65) apply also to smoking marijuana. Smokers have a greater risk of miscarriage, premature delivery, or stillbirth. In mothers who use marijuana, the placenta tends to be smaller and less efficient. Babies may be smaller and less well developed at birth. There appears to be a strong link between marijuana use and hyperactivity and irritability of the newborn. Even the occasional recreational use of marijuana during pregnancy may cause harm and should be avoided.

MEDICATIONS (during pregnancy)

Many medications, even the most ordinary everyday ones that you can buy over the counter, go through the placenta to your baby and might cause harm. For example, aspirin – hardly a dangerous drug under normal circumstances – can be a hazard during pregnancy. Items which were safely prescribed for you when you were not pregnant could cause trouble now. Your doctors have a list of commonly used medications and their possible effects during pregnancy. This list is available for your information. Unless you are sure that the doctors in charge of your obstetrical care recommend a particular medication for you at this time, you should take nothing.

MEDICATIONS (for labor and delivery)

You should discuss with your doctor the issue of medication during labor and delivery well before the day arrives. If you are attending childbirth preparation classes and intend to have an unmedicated labor and delivery, it's important that you and your doctor communicate clearly on your expectations for this experience.

Ask your doctor what would be available if you should require medication during your labor or delivery. Analgesics relieve pain. Anesthetics temporarily deaden sensation including pain. You should feel free to ask about the effects of any of these medications on your birthing experience and on your baby. It's best to talk about this before you go into labor so that there are no misunderstandings. Of course, special circumstances during your labor may present medical reasons for a change in plans.

MISCARRIAGE

Most early (first trimester) miscarriages are nature's way of dealing with a pregnancy resulting from a flawed ovum or sperm, or a pregnancy in which these cells joined incorrectly and could not develop normally. Factors which raise the chances of an early miscarriage include poor nutrition, environmental pollution, smoking, and pelvic inflammatory disease. A miscarriage later in pregnancy may be caused by a structural problem in the womb or cervix.

More than half the women who threaten to miscarry—i.e., show one or more symptoms of a miscarriage—do not lose the pregnancy. However, for those who do lose the pregnancy in the first trimester there is usually nothing that could have been done to change that outcome.

Difficult as it may seem, a woman who miscarries at home should try to save whatever tissue she can. Analysis of the tissue might shed light on what went wrong. If a miscarriage does not completely empty the womb, a brief hospitalization for a D and C might be required.

Miscarriage can be a very difficult emotional experience for both parents. Grieving is appropriate and necessary as well as understandable. (See PREGNANCY LOSS.)

NIPPLE CARE

If you plan to breastfeed your baby, the following steps taken during pregnancy are useful. They may help to prevent nipple soreness when you first start to feed your baby.

- Use water with little or no soap for washing nipples.
- Rub your nipples gently with a terry cloth towel at least twice a day.
- Hold each nipple between your fingers and gently pull and roll it for a minute, twice daily. You may use cream or oil if you wish. If you are allergic to wool, you shouldn't use lanolin, which is made from it.
- Go without a bra, or wear a nursing bra with the flaps down for a little while each day. This exposes your nipples to air and to the gentle friction of your clothing.

If you have flat or inverted (turning inward) nipples, these steps may be more difficult for you, but they can still be done. Special breast shields may be worn to help extend the nipples if they are inverted. Ask your doctor if you need help.

NONSTRESS TEST

If additional information about the condition of your baby is required before delivery, a nonstress test may be recommended. The fetal heart monitor is used for the nonstress test. The baby's heartbeat will be recorded over a period of time, perhaps thirty minutes or more. During this time, you may be asked to indicate whenever you feel the baby move. Variability is looked for in the fetal heartrate as the baby moves. The test may be repeated several times late in your pregnancy. In certain high risk cases, the results of a nonstress test may indicate a need to induce labor.

OXYTOCIN CHALLENGE TEST (STRESS TEST)

The Oxytocin Challenge Test, a stress test, may be used in a high risk late pregnancy as one of the measures to evaluate placental functioning and fetal wellbeing. A stress test stimulates contractions and uses a fetal heart monitor to record the responses of the fetus. This test may be used in suspected cases of postmaturity (overdue baby), or to assist in decision making when there are risk factors such as toxemia, diabetes, hypertension, falling estriol levels, or a small-for-dates baby. The results of the stress test may indicate that the pregnancy should be permitted to continue longer. If not, the results will help the doctor decide whether to induce labor or perform a Caesarean section.

PREGNANCY LOSS

While the majority of pregnancies end successfully for both mother and baby, some do not. You need not (and should not) dwell on the thought that something might go wrong. Your energies are better spent taking the best possible care of yourself and thinking positive thoughts. Nevertheless, it's not inappropriate for expectant parents to give some thought to how they might cope if they do suffer a miscarriage, stillbirth, or neonatal death. Chances are, you won't need the information that follows this paragraph, but we've included it for those who do.

In times past, a pregnancy loss was a virtually unmentionable subject, and the baby's remains were disposed of speedily because it was thought that this would be the easiest for the parents involved. Today, however, parents who lose a child through miscarriage or stillbirth are encouraged to face and acknowledge the loss directly, to talk about it, and to grieve as they would in the death of any other close family member. It is suggested that parents name their baby and participate in a religious or memorial service if they wish. If the baby is fully formed, the parents should see and hold the child. Many of those who do not see and hold their baby express regrets later. If a woman must remain in the hospital after losing a child she should, if at all possible, be treated somewhere other than the maternity/nursery area where she would have to watch happy families with their babies.

Those who suffer a pregnancy loss may find comfort and support from others who themselves have experienced the death of an unborn or very young baby. Your doctor may be able to direct you to a support group in your area. If not, you might contact SHARE, a clearinghouse for support groups for those who have experienced miscarriage or stillbirth. More than 300 groups across the country have registered with SHARE, and there may be one near you. Additional information can be obtained by writing to Sister Jane Marie Lamb, SHARE, St. John's Hospital, 800 East Carpenter Street, Springfield, IL 62769.

PREP

A prep is the shaving of the pubic and perineal area, or just the perineum (mini-prep). Prepping a laboring woman prior to delivery has been a widely practiced hospital routine for decades. The stated purpose for using this procedure is to reduce the risk of infection. However, several studies have demonstrated that the infection rate is lower among those women who have not been shaved. This is probably because the shaving can nick and abrade the skin, thereby leaving openings for bacteria.

A number of doctors and hospitals still order preps routinely because they have always done so. For a woman with very long hair on the perineum, a scissor clip might be used as an alternative to a prep. Prepping is a procedure that many women are choosing to refuse. Discuss your wishes with your doctor in advance.

PREPARED CHILDBIRTH

The major childbirth preparation approaches from which to choose are the Dick-Read natural childbirth method, Bradley's "husband-coached childbirth," the Lamaze method, and Kitzinger's "touch-relaxation" technique. Some childbirth educators offer an eclectic approach which combines aspects of more than one method.

The Dick-Read ("childbirth without fear") method was the pioneering approach to natural childbirth in the U.S. Introduced at a time when fully medicated labors were the norm, and fathers were not permitted in the delivery room, the Dick-Read method originally relied on the medical staff (doctor/midwife/nurse) to provide emotional support to a woman in labor. Now, however, in keeping with current trends, the father is seen as an important member of the team throughout pregnancy and the birthing process.

The Lamaze method, based on Pavlov's theory of conditioned reflex, trains a woman to respond to the stimulus of a contraction with the conditioned response of relaxation rather than the instinctive reponse of tension, fear, and pain. A partner — either the child's father, or some other person with whom the mother feels comfortable — acts as labor coach.

Bradley's method stresses a completely "natural" and unmedicated delivery. The child's father plays an important role during the pregnancy as well as the child's birth. Some of the techniques used in Bradley's husband-coached childbirth were derived from observations of the instinctive behavior of animals during labor and delivery.

Kitzinger's method of childbirth preparation, which is very popular in England, places strong emphasis on the emotional and psychological aspects of childbearing as well as on body awareness and relaxation techniques.

The type of classes you attend will, of course, depend on what is convenient and available for you as well as which approach you favor. Even if you think that your preference leans toward an unprepared, medicated labor and delivery, classes are recommended. The information gained will help you participate in your baby's birth in the way that is best for both of you.

If at all possible, you and your partner should plan to attend a series of childbirth preparation classes. Most expectant parents begin classes in the seventh month, although it's a good idea to sign up earlier. Your doctor's office can direct you to classes available in your area.

Prepared Childbirth Classes	
Date and Time	**Teacher – Topic**

In childbirth preparation classes you will learn facts about labor and delivery that will help you to deal with it. You will learn to work with your body using special relaxing, controlled breathing, and pushing techniques. Your partner will learn how to assist you.

If your partner can not or will not attend classes, it's still a good idea for you to go. What you learn will help you to work with the nurses and doctor during your labor and delivery.

Do not avoid classes because you fear that you might "fail." No amount of preparation will guarantee that your labor and delivery will go exactly as expected. Attending classes does not commit you to doing things in a particular way once the time comes. The goal of classes is meaningful participation as well as performance. What you learn will increase the choices available to you.

Rh-NEGATIVE MOTHERS

The blood test done early in pregnancy indicates whether or not a mother's blood contains the Rh factor. If it does, the blood is described as Rh Positive (Rh+). If not, it is called Rh Negative (Rh−). If your blood is Rh Negative, and your baby's father has Rh Positive blood, the child may inherit the Rh factor from him and be Rh+ too. This would make your blood incompatible with that of your baby. As a result, your body may produce antibodies to protect itself from this "foreign substance." The antibodies may be strong enough to attack the Rh+ blood of a child in a future pregnancy.

Fortunately, there is now a solution to the problem of an Rh− mother and an Rh+ baby. Within 72 hours of delivery (or miscarriage or abortion) of an Rh+ child, the mother must receive an injection of Rh immune globulin (called RhoGAM). This protects future unborn children by preventing antibodies from forming in the mother's blood.

In a small number of Rh− women, antibodies may be produced during pregnancy as well as after delivery. An injection of RhoGAM during week 28 of the pregnancy can prevent this problem. Because there is no way to predict in advance which cases will need this treatment, many physicians recommend that all Rh− women receive RhoGAM during pregnancy as a precaution. This procedure is safe for both mother and fetus. Another dose of RhoGAM after delivery is required if the baby has Rh+ blood.

If you are Rh+, there is no need for you to worry about any of this. If you and the baby's father are both Rh−, there is also no need for concern. The problem only arises with an Rh− mother and an Rh+ baby.

ROOMING-IN

Some hospitals have rooming-in facilities which permit a mother to keep her newborn baby right in the room with her instead of returning the child to the nursery after feedings. Many mothers enjoy the opportunity to take full care of the new baby right away. Others would prefer to rest completely the first few days after delivery.

If rooming-in appeals to you, be sure to ask about it. It usually costs a bit more, and in some hospitals the facilities are limited and available on a first-come, first-served basis. The type of rooming-in may vary from one hospital to another. Some facilities permit the baby to remain in the mother's room around the clock, both day and night. Others return the baby to the nursery at night. If having your baby with you all the time right from the start is especially important to you, this might influence your choice of birth setting.

RUBELLA

A woman who develops rubella (German measles) during the first three months of pregnancy has as great as a 50-50 chance of having a baby with severe problems such as brain damage, blindness, deafness, or heart and circulatory system defects. At your initial prenatal visit to your doctor, your blood was probably tested to find your level of immunity to rubella. If you have never had rubella and you are not immune, be extra careful to avoid being near anyone with an active case of the disease. Fortunately, as more and more preschool children are routinely immunized, the occurrence of rubella is becoming increasingly rare. Nevertheless, caution is in order. If you think you may have been exposed to rubella (or any other contagious disease) consult your physician.

SAUNAS AND HOT TUBS

The use of saunas or hot tubs is not recommended during pregnancy. The extreme temperatures can cause complications for you as well as damage to your developing baby. Even when you are taking a regular tub bath, you should be careful that the temperature of the water is not higher than 100 degrees. Especially during the first three months, soaking in very hot water can result in fetal damage.

SIBLING PARTICIPATION

Some families wish their children to be present at the birth of a new family member. Many alternative birth centers and some hospitals do permit siblings to be present at delivery. This practice, however, may not be appropriate or comfortable for many families, and you needn't feel that you are depriving your older children of an essential experience if you decide to leave them home. Here are some points to keep in mind if you do plan to have your other children with you during labor and delivery.

- Make sure that the children are prepared for the experience and really want to be there. Your decision to have them present should meet their needs as well as your own.
- A responsible adult who is not your labor coach/companion should accompany each child and be prepared to leave the scene with him or her if necessary.
- Make arrangements for sibling participation in advance with your doctor or midwife. Don't count on being able to show up in labor at a local hospital with an unannounced family entourage and have everything go according to your wishes. If the presence of your other children at delivery is very important to you, this may influence your choice of birth setting.

Most hospitals will make some provision for your children to visit their mother and new brother or sister after the baby is born. Find out ahead of time what procedures are followed in the place where you plan to give birth. Most families find that a sibling visit to the nursery and a chance for children to see their mother are worth the effort.

SMOKING

Many recent studies point to the conclusion that smoking during pregnancy can be very harmful to your unborn child. Cigarette smoke introduces carbon monoxide, nicotine, and tar to your bloodstream. This cuts down on available oxygen for your baby and it reduces the ability of the placenta to pass on nutrients and to get rid of

Warning: The Surgeon General Has Determined That Cigarette Smoking Is Dangerous to Your Health. Smoking During Pregnancy Can Cause Fetal Damage.

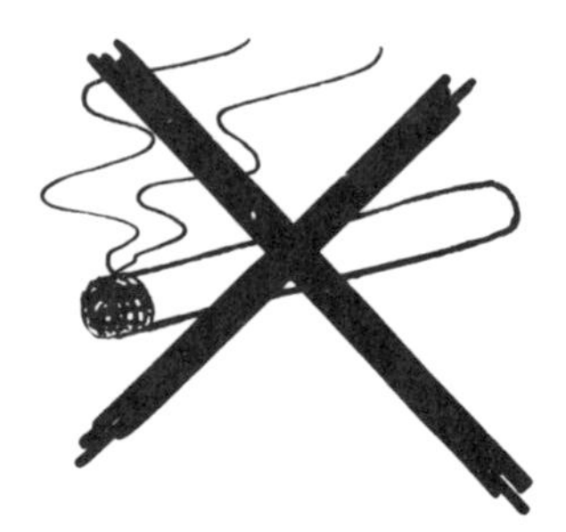

wastes. The body of someone who smokes is less able to use vitamins such as B_{12} and C, and the baby is shortchanged in this way as well.

The baby of a mother who smokes is likely to be smaller and less well developed at birth. Smoking mothers tend to have more frequent miscarriages, premature deliveries, and stillbirths than women who do not smoke. The babies of smokers are more vulnerable to respiratory problems and diseases of early infancy and are at greater risk of dying in infancy. Smoking is not good for you or your baby. If you have been unable to stop smoking for your own sake, perhaps the welfare of your unborn child will be the extra encouragement you need to do it now.

SPORTS

Unless you're a surfer, diver, or water skier, you may continue all your customary athletic activities during pregnancy. It's best to stay away from violent water sports in which a fall or pounding surf could force water up your vagina, but most other sports are fine. You need limit yourself only when **you** notice discomfort beyond what is normal for you. The best guideline to follow is common sense.

To avoid the further straining of joints already strained by your pregnancy, warm up slowly and thoroughly before engaging in strenuous activity. As your pregnancy progresses and your shape changes, you'll have to make adjustments to accommodate your changing center of balance and new size.

Stay with those physical activities to which your body was accustomed prior to your pregnancy. This is not the time to take up a new sport, especially one in which your lack of skill could add to the risk. For example, horseback riding or skiing might be fine for you if that has been a part of your regular routine up to now, but don't get on a horse or skis if you've never done it before.

Most people are able to do whatever they have been used to doing—jogging, biking, hiking, tennis, swimming, riding, or whatever—as long as they feel up to it. Unless there is some special problem with your pregnancy, you can continue most sports as long as you wish. If you would like some specific guidance about appropriate activities for you, feel free to ask your doctor. What is comfortable for one person is quite unsuitable for another so, within reason, you're probably the best judge of what's best for you.

TAMPONS

Most women find that a mini-pad provides enough protection from the common vaginal discharge experienced during pregnancy. If you do not find a pad comfortable and feel that you must use a tampon, check with your doctor. For any tampon user, pregnant or not, we suggest the following guidelines:

(1) Do not use tampons containing perfume or deodorant.
(2) Do not use any tampon that has been chemically treated to increase absorbency.
(3) Tampons with cardboard applicators or those requiring no applicator may be a safer choice because plastic applicators can cut you and leave openings for bacteria.
(4) Change the tampon frequently, and be sure your hands are clean before you do so. It's best not to leave a tampon in longer than four hours.

TOXEMIA OF PREGNANCY

Toxemia of pregnancy is a disease which can be very dangerous for a pregnant woman and her baby. Symptoms of the disease include swelling of body tissues with rapid weight gain, high blood pressure, and protein (albumin) in the urine. Any two of these symptoms in combination indicate that a serious problem may be developing.

Despite much research on the subject, doctors do not agree on the exact cause of toxemia of pregnancy. They do agree, however, that the best cure is prevention. In its mild or early stages, toxemia can be controlled. In cases where treatment is lacking or unsuccessful, the symptoms get more severe as time goes on. A severely toxemic mother is in danger of having convulsions (eclampsia) which could be fatal to her or her baby. Blood flow through the placenta is decreased with toxemia and this causes the baby to suffer. Babies of toxemic mothers tend to be small in relation to the length of time they are carried. They have a greater chance of being stillborn.

Toxemia is more likely to occur in women whose diets are low in protein, high in salt, or both. Making sure that the diet includes enough protein and the B vitamins to help the body use protein is important. Salt restrictions may be ordered. If so, watch out for surprise sources of sodium (salt) such as cold cuts, frozen or canned vegetables, diet sodas or Chinese foods. Read labels carefully.

Bed rest is often prescribed to keep the symptoms of toxemia under control. Elevating the feet may help somewhat. One of the problems with controlling toxemia is that the mother feels little or no discomfort during the early stages of the disease. She may not take the doctor's warning seriously until it's too late. If you are advised that you are developing symptoms of toxemia, it's very important to follow the doctor's suggestions even if you think you feel all right. Your life and your baby's could depend on it.

PREVENT TOXEMIA

Your daily diet should contain:

- plenty of protein
- enough B Vitamins
- not too much salt

If your doctor tells you to rest with your feet up, DO IT, even if you're sure you feel fine.

TOXIC SUBSTANCES

Although you should try to avoid unnecessary contact with toxic substances in your environment at all times, this is especially important during pregnancy. It may surprise you to learn that some of the products you use routinely are potentially hazardous. Read labels carefully.

- Use household cleaners (especially those that produce fumes) only in well ventilated areas. Avoid unnecessary exposure to cleaning substances such as dusting sprays or bathroom tile cleaners.
- Avoid the use of aerosol containers whenever possible, and never use an aerosol can in a poorly ventilated place. If you shop carefully, you'll probably find that most of the products you would buy in a spray can have a non-aerosol alternative.
- Minimize any contact with insecticides, pesticides, weed killers, and similar substances in your home or garden. If any of these items must be used, it's best to let someone else do the work.

- No matter how eager you might be to refinish baby furniture or paint your baby's room, you should probably not use paint removers or solvents while you are pregnant. If you must, choose the least volatile you can find, and be sure you work in a well-ventilated place. Latex-base paints are safer for you to use than oil base paints, but you'll be safer letting someone else do the painting.
- Be cautious about personal items such as cosmetics, permanent wave solutions, and hair dyes. Read ingredients carefully. Stay away from products containing lead, mercury, or arsenic.

TOXOPLASMOSIS

Toxoplasmosis is a flulike illness caused by protozoa. The disease in an adult is often so mild that it passes virtually unnoticed, but it can be extremely harmful—even fatal—for a fetus. When contracted by a pregnant woman, toxoplasmosis can result in severe brain or liver damage for her unborn child. Another effect toxoplasmosis may have on a fetus is damage to the retina of the eye, resulting in severe visual impairment or blindness. These visual handicaps may show up immediately in an affected infant, or they may not develop until years later, but any child who contracts toxoplasmosis in the womb is at risk for visual problems.

Cats and raw meat are the two common sources of toxoplasma parasites. Fortunately, it's easy to minimize your chances of exposure.

- If you have a cat you absolutely can't part with, get someone else to clean the litter box. Avoid any contact whatsoever with cat feces.
- While you are pregnant, the meat you eat should be thoroughly cooked. Leave steak tartare or very rare hamburgers off your menu until after your baby is born.

TRAVEL

Travel during pregnancy is fine. Being pregnant is not a reason to keep you home if there's somewhere you want to go.

Avoid sitting still for long periods in a car, bus, plane, or train. Stretch your body, arms, and legs every hour or so. Get up and walk about for a few minutes each hour or hour and a half. If you are driving, you must be sure to remember to pull over and get a bit of exercise. This will help prevent slowdown of your circulation and possible clot formation.

If you plan to travel by air while you are pregnant, there are a number of things to keep in mind.

- You'll probably feel better if you eat and drink sensibly en route. You don't have to eat something just because a flight attendant puts it in front of you. Many airlines permit you to order special meals (e.g., vegetarian, low salt, a sandwich) when you make the reservation. See what's available.
- Seats by a door or bulkhead generally have more room. Remember that you will be getting up to move around and to use the lavatory more than you might at other times.
- Some airlines permit a pregnant passenger to skip the electronic security check and be checked by a person instead. Ask.
- Fasten the seatbelt loosely — across your lap and under your protruding abdomen.

- While seated, try to elevate your feet if you can. Pillows placed at the small of your back may make you more comfortable.
- Your feet and legs may swell more than usual during a long flight. It's best not to remove your shoes, because you might have trouble putting them back on when you land.

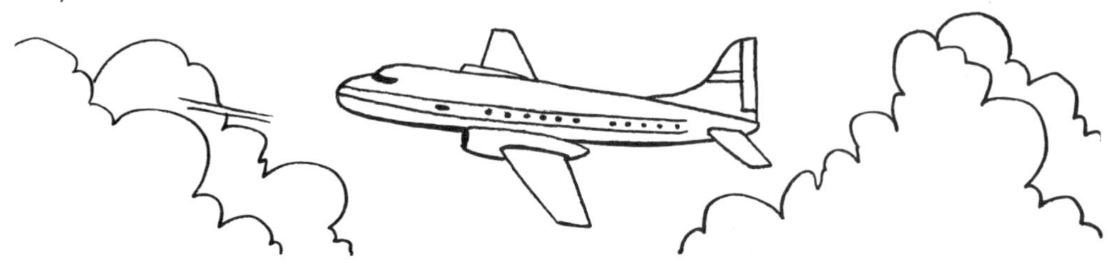

The potential hazards of flying — accident, hijacking, equipment failure — are generally the same whether or not a passenger is pregnant. One exception to this would be a rapid change in cabin pressure at high altitudes. The immediate use of supplemental oxygen would be extremely important for a pregnant woman. And, a severe pressure change could result in ruptured membranes. However, the chances of such an equipment failure on modern commercial jets are very small indeed, and should be considered in light of the need to travel and the convenience of flying.

If you are visibly pregnant, you should check with the airline you'll be using to find out any special regulations for flying while pregnant. The rules vary greatly from one airline to another. Some airlines restrict travel during the week before the due date. Others ban it for the last month or even two. Some require a doctor's certificate. Others take your word for it. An overcautious airline employee may not let you board if you appear to be close to delivery. This can happen even if you and your doctor think travel at that time is fine. It's best to check on these things before you make final plans for a trip. The only way you can be sure of an airline's policy is to call and ask.

As your due date nears, unnecessary travel that involves great distances is not recommended because labor may begin in an inconvenient place.

TWINS

Twins occur about once in ninety births. Identical twins are from a single fertilized ovum which splits completely very early in pregnancy and then develops into two babies. Fraternal twins develop from two different fertilized eggs. Because they have identical chromosome distribution, identical twins have the same sex, blood type, appearance, and other inherited characteristics. Fraternal twins, on the other hand, may be as alike or as different as any two children of the same parents.

If your doctor finds that your uterus is increasing in size more rapidly than would be expected, a multiple pregnancy may be the reason. Locating two separate fetal heartbeats could confirm the diagnosis. A sonogram can provide definite information about the number of babies a woman is carrying.

If you are having more than one baby, you may notice some of the possible discomforts of pregnancy more strongly than someone who is having only one child. Paying close attention to the suggestions for coping with bodily changes, pages 15 to 24, may be helpful. Ask your doctor if there are any modifications to these suggestions for your particular situation.

Premature delivery is a frequent complication associated with multiple births. Because of this, a woman known to be carrying twins might need extra rest during the last three months of pregnancy. If this is necessary in your case, your doctor will advise you.

ULTRASOUND

Ultrasonography is a diagnostic technique which uses high frequency sound waves. Ultrasound can provide pictures of soft tissues in considerable detail. Real-time is a continuous ultrasound that can be seen on a TV monitor. It shows motion, and can also be recorded in still frames using a polaroid camera.

An ultrasound test, or sonogram as it is commonly called, is used for a number of different purposes. It can be used to determine the age and the size of the fetus, and one may be ordered in mid-pregnancy if there is some question about the actual due date. A sonogram can show the location of the placenta, the presence of certain abnormalities, and multiple births. In some cases, a sonogram may also indicate the sex of the fetus.

If you have amniocentesis, a sonogram will be done to locate the precise location of the fetus and the placenta, so the physician knows exactly where to insert the needle to withdraw amniotic fluid.

Ultrasound is a useful diagnostic technique and should be employed when the information it can obtain is medically needed. There are no known harmful effects to mother or baby. However, the long term effects of the use of ultrasound have not been studied and are not known at this time. Routine or unnecessary sonograms should be avoided. If a sonogram is recommended for you, feel free to ask any questions you might have about the indications for it or the interpretation of the results.

VBAC (VAGINAL BIRTH AFTER CAESAREAN)

Until recently, any woman who had a baby by Caesarean section could count on having future children that way as well. Now the practice of routine repeat Caesareans is changing, as more and more women are demanding an opportunity to attempt VBAC (pronounced Vee-back), and more and more doctors are willing to give them that chance.

If your previous Caesarean used a low horizontal uterine incision, a vaginal delivery may be as safe for your baby as a repeat Caesarean, and it may be even safer for you. Here are some suggestions to help you achieve a vaginal birth after Caesarean, if at all possible for your particular circumstances.

- Find a supportive obstetrician who is willing to attempt VBAC and who is actively committed to helping you succeed.
- Be sure to attend childbirth preparation classes. Try to find an instructor who provides information and supportive instruction on VBAC.
- Consider hiring a midwife or monitrice to be with you in labor, especially if your obstetrician requires VBAC candidates to come to the hospital in early labor. The close personal support of a birth attendant who focuses on delivery as a normal process rather than a medical problem can help get you safely through a longer trial of labor than you might be able to manage on your own.

Even if you are well prepared and highly motivated, and your birth attendants are supportive, it's possible that you'll require a repeat Caesarean anyway. There may be a new reason unrelated to the first Caesarean, or a recurrence of the previous cause. If this should occur, remember it doesn't mean you have failed. It simply means that a medical decision was made at the time of need, rather than months earlier in anticipation of something that might never have happened.

VENEREAL DISEASE

Sexually transmitted (venereal) diseases are a serious health problem in today's world. Certain of these diseases can cause severe harm or even death to a developing fetus. It's important for a pregnant woman who suspects she might have been infected to tell her doctor immediately so that the disease can be identified and treatment started.

A routine blood test done during an early prenatal visit to the doctor or clinic checks for syphilis, a disease which can cause a variety of defects as well as death of an unborn child. Some syphilis-related disorders may not appear until many years later. If the routine blood test is positive, further testing is done to see what treatment is required. If identified promptly, syphilis can usually be cured completely.

If a woman has gonorrhea at the time of labor and delivery, this can infect the baby during passage through the birth canal and cause blindness. Most states require that medication (e.g., antibiotic ointment or silver nitrate drops) be applied to the baby's eyes soon after birth to prevent infection. Gonorrhea is curable and can be treated with antibiotics.

Herpes virus (Type 2) is becoming increasingly common. During its active stage, this virus causes painful sores on the genitals. There is no known cure for genital herpes at this time, although the symptoms can be controlled and some relief provided.

A pregnant woman who carries the herpes virus may be more likely to miscarry, give birth prematurely, or have a low birthweight baby. Careful medical management of pregnancy and delivery for a woman with herpes is especially important to help minimize the potential risks to the baby. Because a newborn who contracts herpes in the birth canal may die or be severely handicapped, delivery by Caesarean section is indicated for a mother with an active case of genital herpes.

To help prevent the spread of herpes, avoid oral sex if you or your partner have cold sores or fever blisters. The sores or blisters contain the active virus, and you should wash your hands carefully before any genital contact. It is possible for oral herpes virus (Type 1),which causes sores around the mouth,to cause sores on the genitals as well. A person with an active case of oral herpes should use paper plates and disposable utensils until the sores have healed. The herpes virus can survive on a household surface long enough to reinfect a person. Even though infection in this way is very unlikely, a strong chlorine bleach solution or other recommended disinfectant should be used in the laundry and to clean surfaces.

If you suspect that you might have a venereal disease, be sure to tell your doctor or other health care provider. Don't let embarrassment keep you from getting help when you need it. Your health and your baby's life may depend on it.

WEIGHT

During your pregnancy a weight gain of 24 to 30 pounds is normal. Unless your doctor tells you otherwise, this is what you should aim for. If you are eating nutritious food, your gain is not fat. Most of this weight can be lost within two to six weeks after you give birth.

The material on nutrition during pregnancy, pages 31 to 46, describes what foods you should be eating. Do not diet to lose weight while you are pregnant. Your baby and your hard-working body need the recommended calories. A typical weight gain of 24 pounds during pregnancy would be distributed as follows: first 3 months—about 3 pounds; second three months—about 10 pounds; last three months—about 11 pounds.

For a typical mother who eats wisely during pregnancy, here's what the recommended 24 pound gain might include.

BABY	7-1/2 pounds	BLOOD	3-1/2 pounds
PLACENTA	1-1/2 pounds	OTHER FLUID	2-3/4 pounds
AMNIOTIC FLUID	2 pounds	UTERUS	2-1/2 pounds
BREAST TISSUE	1 pound	OTHER	3-1/4 pounds

Use the following chart to keep track of your weight gain.

Date – Weight	**Date – Weight**	**Date – Weight**	**Date – Weight**

X-RAYS

While you are pregnant, you should avoid X-rays if at all possible. Routine diagnostic X-rays, such as those for nonessential dental work, should be postponed until after your baby is born. If an emergency or a medical condition unrelated to your pregnancy should require you to have an X-ray, it's important that the prescribing physician and radiology staff know you are pregnant so that appropriate precautions can be taken in administering the procedure.

BOOKS FOR YOUR INFORMATION

As you work with your doctor or midwife and prepared childbirth instructor throughout your pregnancy, you'll probably find that WHILE WAITING contains the basic information you need on topics most important to your health care. For further reading about pregnancy, childbirth, and newborn baby care, additional titles are suggested below.

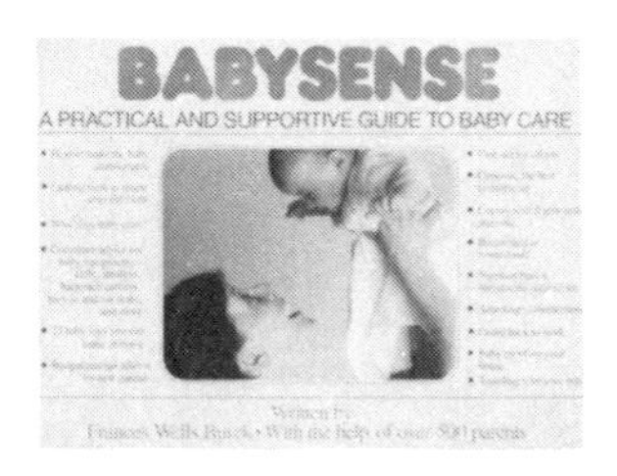

Babysense: A Practical and Supportive Guide to Baby Care
Frances Wells Burck (St. Martin's Press, New York: 1979)
A reassuring guide for baby care during the first year, along with suggestions for a mother's postpartum recovery. More than 500 parents contributed suggestions to this practical book.

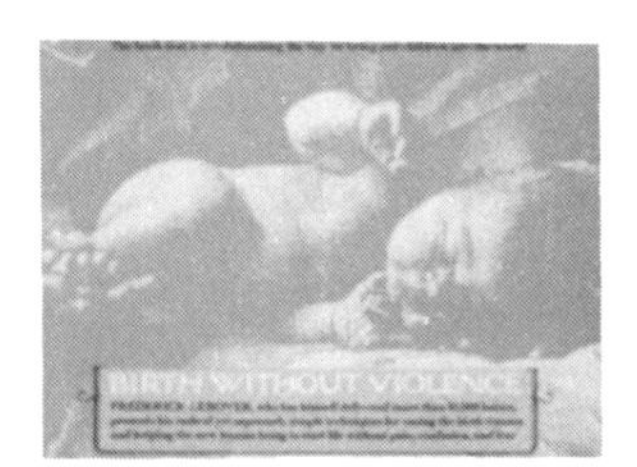

Birth Without Violence
Frederick Leboyer, M.D. (Alfred A. Knopf, Inc., New York: 1975)
Beautifully written text and fine photographs focus on the baby's needs and feelings during the birth process. Leboyer makes a powerful case which is worth reading even if you don't entirely agree with his ideas or methods.

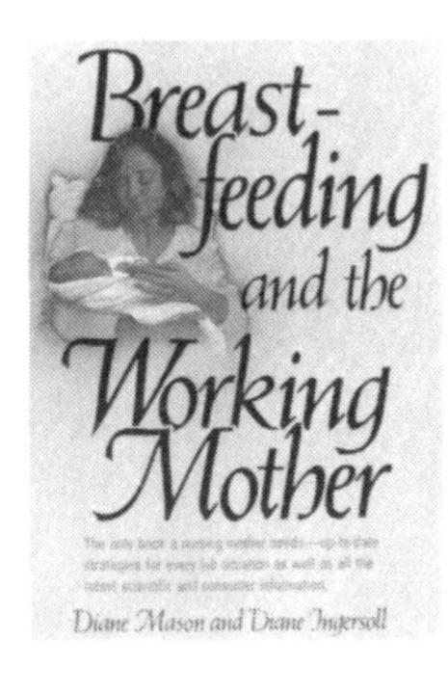

Breastfeeding and the Working Mother
Diane Mason and Diane Ingersoll (St. Martin's Press, New York: 1986)
A complete handbook for mothers who want to breastfeed and continue working. Covers breastfeeding and provides practical tips for mothers in every conceivable job situation—full-time, part-time, travel, meetings. The book also covers nursing dress, equipment, and legal rights. A useful guide whether or not you plan to work outside the home.

Caring for Your Unborn Child
Ronald E. Gots, M.D., Ph.D., and Barbara A. Gots, M.D. (Bantam Books, New York: 1979)
Describes the effects of a mother's diet, environment, and personal habits on a baby's development from conception to birth, and identifies harmful substances to avoid.

A Child Is Born
Lennart Nilsson (Delacorte Press/Seymour Lawrence, New York: 1977)
An unusual and worthwhile (although costly) addition to any home library. Fascinating photographs of prenatal life provide information and help to communicate a sense of the mystery and beauty of a new life from the moment of conception.

Childbirth Without Fear: The Principles and Practices of Natural Childbirth
Grantly Dick-Read (Harper and Row Publishers, New York: 1974)
The pioneer in introducing childbirth education and natural childbirth methods to the United States. The approach has evolved with changing trends, and now actively involves the father as a major source of emotional support.

The Complete Book of Pregnancy and Childbirth
Sheila Kitzinger (Alfred A. Knopf, Inc., New York: 1980)
Comprehensive, beautifully written and illustrated, and definitely one of the best books we've seen. This book can help you develop awareness and understanding of the childbearing process so you can fully and actively participate in the experience in the most joyful and satisfying way for yourself, your partner, and your baby.

Easing Labor Pain
Adrienne B. Lieberman (Doubleday & Co., Inc., Garden City, New York: 1987)
A handbook of strategies to deal with labor pain. This supportive book covers a wide range of possibilities—from acupuncture and biofeedback to Lamaze to medical intervention, and can help you choose the birthing plan that is best for you.

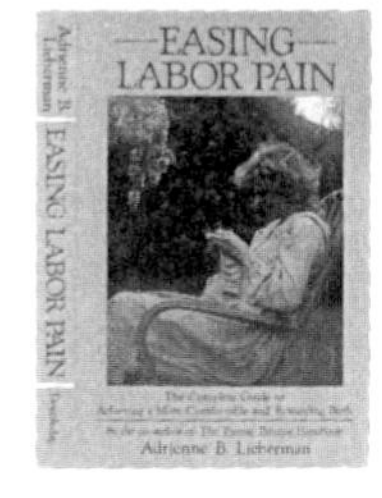

Essential Exercises for the Childbearing Year
Elizabeth Noble (Houghton Mifflin Company, Boston: 1982)
A comprehensive collection of exercises for fitness during pregnancy and a rapid postpartum recovery. Drawings and diagrams illustrate the specific instructions.

The Experience of Childbirth (Fourth Revised Edition)
Sheila Kitzinger (Penguin Books, New York: 1978)
A guide to Kitzinger's touch-relaxation method of prepared childbirth. This book deals with the emotional as well as the physical aspects of childbearing.

The Facts of Life
Jonathan Miller and David Pelham (Viking Penguin, Inc., New York: 1984)
An unusual and fascinating volume about human reproduction. Its intricate three-dimensional illustrations move or pop up to demonstrate with amazing clarity how conception, prenatal development, and birth occur.

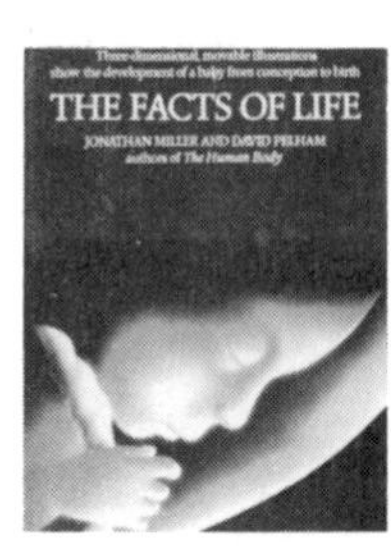

Giving Birth
Adrienne B. Lieberman (St. Martin's Press, New York: 1987)
A practical and reassuring guide to what happens during labor and birth. Includes first-person accounts from twelve different couples, and excellent suggestions to prepare you for the unexpected as well as choices you can make in advance.

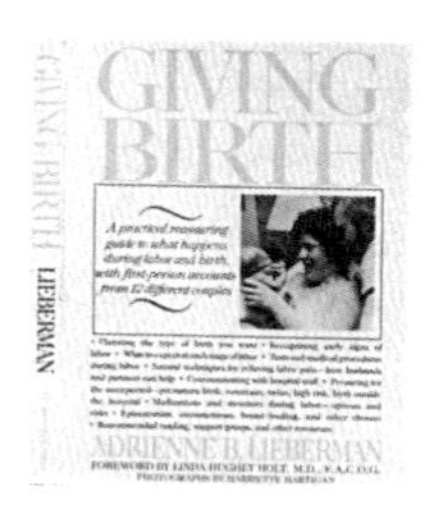

A Good Birth, A Safe Birth
Diana Korte and Roberta Scaer (Bantam Books, New York: 1984)
Detailed information about today's trends in childbirth and the options available. This consumer-oriented volume can help you achieve the childbearing experience you wish in a hospital setting. Excellent bibliography and list of resources.

Having a Baby: A Complete Guide for the Mother-to-Be
Eric Trimmer, M.B., B.S., M.R.C.G.P. (St. Martin's Press, New York: 1981)
Contains the nine-month diary of a pregnant woman illustrated with color photographs, and a detailed presentation of information about pregnancy, delivery, and care of the newborn baby, along with suggestions for personal health care.

Husband-Coached Childbirth (Third Edition)
Robert A. Bradley (Harper and Row Publishers, New York: 1981)
Describes Bradley's method of prepared childbirth in which the father's participation throughout pregnancy and birth is stressed. Bradley's enthusiasm for this natural, non-medicated, family-centered approach is evident in his writing.

Jane Fonda's Workout Book for Pregnancy, Birth, and Recovery
Femmy DeLyser (Simon and Schuster, New York: 1982)
A comprehensive exercise program for pregnancy and after. This volume is expensive, so look before you buy, to make sure it meets your needs. The program is also available on video cassette for those who prefer to listen and watch instead of read.

Nourishing Your Unborn Child
Phyllis S. Williams, R.N. (Avon Books, New York: 1982)
A useful source of detailed information on nutrition during pregnancy. It includes more than 150 pages of menus and recipes.

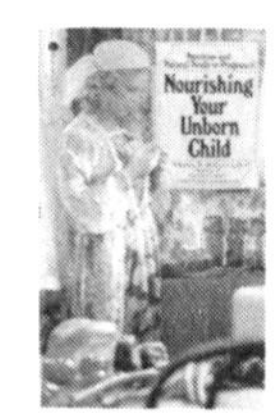

Painless Childbirth: The Lamaze Method
Fernand Lamaze (Pocket Books, New York: 1965)
A reference for those interested in the historical and theoretical background of the Lamaze method. For the practical application of these techniques see the books by Donna and Roger Ewy or Elizabeth Bing.

The Parents' Guide to Raising Twins
Elizabeth Friedrich and Cherry Rowland (St. Martin's Press, New York: 1984)
A useful book for those who suspect or know they are having more than one. The authors, both mothers of twins, write from personal experience as well as other research.

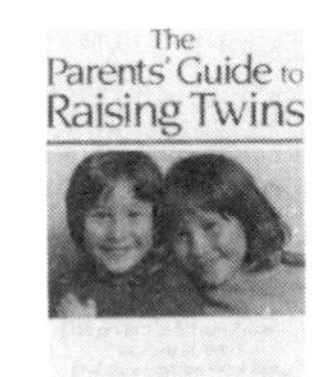

Pregnancy After 35
Carole Spearin McCauley (Pocket Books, New York: 1978)
A comprehensive guide to prenatal care especially for women over 35, but useful for others as well. This book contains sections on genetic counseling and on single parenting.

The Premature Baby Book: A Parents' Guide to Coping and Caring in the First Years
Helen Harrison, with Ann Kositsky, R.N. (St. Martin's Press, New York: 1983)
Contains a wealth of medical and practical information and support for parents of a premature baby. If your waiting ended significantly sooner than you had anticipated, this book is a must.

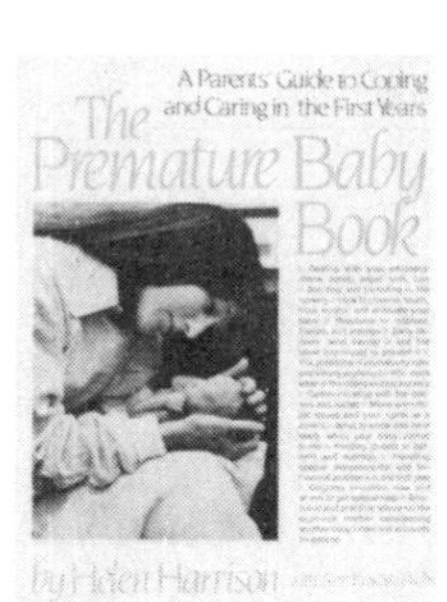

Preparation for Childbirth: A Lamaze Guide
Donna and Roger Ewy (New American Library, New York: 1982)
Presents detailed directions for breathing, relaxing, and conditioning exercises in preparation for childbirth and includes clear instructions for the labor coach as well as for the mother.

Six Practical Lessons for an Easier Childbirth
Elizabeth Bing (Bantam Books, New York: 1982)
A book on the Lamaze method which presents the techniques and practice exercises in detail. The author pioneered in introducing the method in the United States.

Suzy Prudden's Pregnancy and Back-to-Shape Exercise Program
Suzy Prudden and Jeffrey Sussman (Workman Press, New York: 1980)
A fine collection of exercises for pregnancy and postpartum, including starter exercises for the newborn. The directions for each exercise are clear and concise. Excellent photographs illustrate the text.

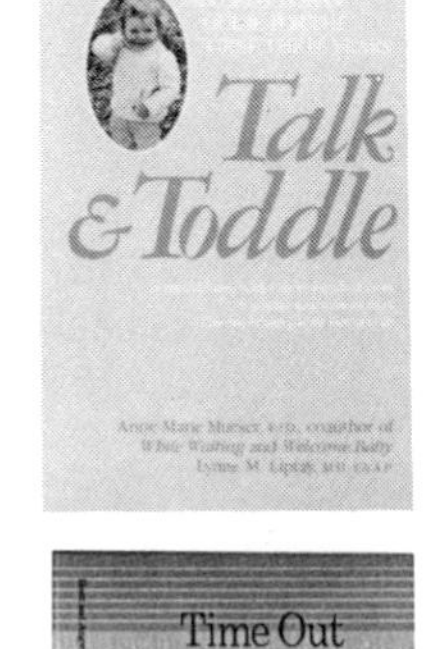

Talk and Toddle: A Commonsense Guide for the First Three Years
Anne Marie Mueser, Ed.D., and Lynne M. Liptay, M.D. (St. Martin's Press, New York: 1983)
Before long your newborn will be a mobile baby and then a toddler. This book is designed to help you cope with these demanding and exciting early years. The many topics of concern to a toddler's parents are alphabetically arranged for easy references.

Time Out for Motherhood
Lucy Scott, Ph.D., and Meredith Joan Angwin (Jeremy P. Tarcher, Inc., Los Angeles: 1986)
A useful guide to the financial, emotional, and career aspects of combining motherhood with work outside the home.

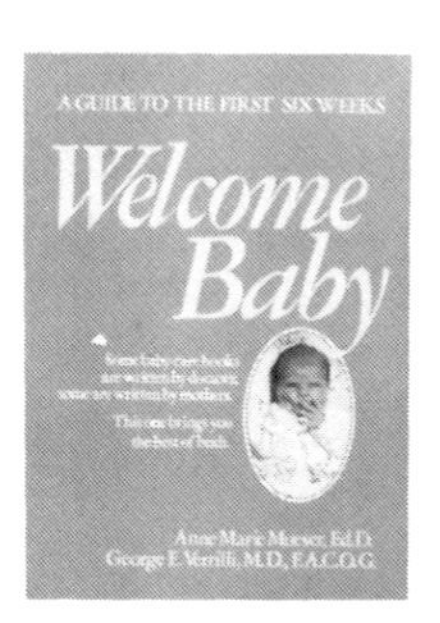

Welcome Baby: A Guide to the First Six Weeks
Anne Marie Mueser, Ed.D., and George E. Verrilli, M.D. (St. Martin's Press, New York: 1982)
Contains numerous helpful suggestions for the busy days and weeks after your new baby's arrival. This companion volume to *While Waiting* is presented in the same easy-to-read style and format.

SOME QUESTIONS...WHILE WAITING

Many women have questions and concerns about labor and delivery. This is especially true for a first baby. It's important to feel free to ask any questions you might have, and this list is designed to help you do that. Circle the ? next to each question you would like to discuss with your doctor. Mark with an X each question which has already been answered or which does not interest you. Space is provided for notes and other questions you might have.

?	How can I tell if I am high risk? If I am, what should I be doing differently? What extra precautions will be taken by my medical team?
?	What are the chances that I will need a Caesarean delivery? How can I prepare for this? Can my partner remain with me?
?	If I have previously had a Caesarean, will I be permitted to labor and attempt a vaginal delivery this time?
?	If I prepare for an unmedicated delivery, do I have the option of changing my mind?
?	If I prefer not to be medicated, how can I be sure that the hospital staff will respect my wishes?
?	If I require medication during labor or delivery, what will be available to me? How will this affect the baby? How will it alter my birthing experience?
?	In preparing me for delivery, will an enema and/or pubic shave be ordered or suggested? If I choose not to have these procedures, how can this be arranged?
?	Will I be required to have an I-V during labor as a matter of routine? In the absence of any specific medical indications for an I-V, may I choose to refuse this intervention?
?	If my membranes do not rupture spontaneously before or during early labor, will an amniotomy be required? If so, why? When might this be done? May I choose not to have this procedure?

?	Will my labor be monitored electronically? What alternatives do I have if I choose not to be monitored in this way?
?	May I hire a monitrice (private obstetrical nurse) to attend me during my labor and delivery?
?	Will I be permitted to walk around during labor? Will I be encouraged to labor and deliver in the position I find most comfortable?
?	May I invite someone in addition to my support partner to be with me in labor and delivery? What about friends or my other children?
?	What is a forceps delivery? Why is this sometimes necessary?
?	Must an episiotomy be done routinely? What can we do to reduce the need for this procedure?
?	What arrangements, if any, must be made in advance for the Leboyer approach to a nonviolent birth?
?	What is bonding? Are there any special preparations I should make for this? How much time will I be able to spend with my baby in the delivery room?
?	Will I be permitted to nurse my baby immediately after delivery if I wish?
?	What routine medical procedures will be required for my baby immediately after birth? May I choose to delay or modify these routines?
?	How can I choose a pediatrician who will support me in the early experiences I wish for my baby and myself as a family?

?	If all goes well, how soon may I leave the hospital after my baby is born?
?	
?	
?	
?	

Section Five

LABOR AND DELIVERY

Pre-Term Labor: What if Labor Starts Too Soon? What Are Warning Signals? What Can Your Healthcare Team Do? / When the Baby is Overdue: How Long is Too Long? What Can Be Done? / Signs of Labor: Contractions, Rupture of Membranes, "Show" / The Waiting Is Over: When Should We Call the Doctor or Midwife? When Should We Leave for the Hospital? / What to Bring / The Hospital Admissions Office / What Happens Next? / Guidelines for Labor and Delivery / First Stage of Labor / Second Stage of Labor / Third Stage of Labor / Apgar Rating / Baby Care (delivery room) / Additional Medical Procedures / Circumcision / Baby Care (nursery) / Baby's Doctor / Naming Your Baby / Your Care After Delivery / Hospital Stay

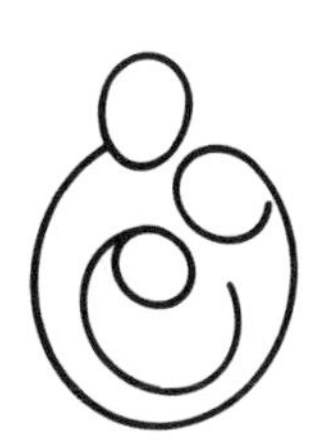

PRE-TERM LABOR

What If Labor Starts Too Soon?

Call your doctor immediately if you think that you are experienceing any of the signs of labor sooner than you think you should. Be alert to the warning signals of pregnancy complications , and don't be afraid to call if you feel something is not right. If you are truly in premature labor, it's important to receive medical attention without delay. If you are mistaken, the extra phone call will cause no harm.

What Are Warning Signals for Pre-Term Labor?

For some women, backache and pelvic discomfort may be normal experiences of pregnancy. However, persistent or rhythmic low back or pelvic pressure, especially if it feels different from what you've felt up to now, may be a warning signal. Cramps—either like those of a menstrual period, or intestinal cramps with or without diarrhea—may signal a complication. An increase or change in vaginal discharge, especially if the discharge is clear and watery or tinged with blood, should be reported promptly.

What Can Your Healthcare Team Do?

Once pre-term labor has begun, it may not be possible to stop the process. However, there are measures—including use of one or more labor-stopping drugs—which may be effective if employed soon enough. If pre-term labor is effectively halted, bed rest and complete relaxation will be ordered to delay the recurrence of labor as long as possible. If labor can be delayed, a drug to hasten the baby's lung development may be administered.

If you experience premature labor, you may be directed to a nearby hospital with neonatal care facilities, even if that's not the place you had planned to deliver. If your pre-term labor can't be stopped, it's important that your premature infant be in a facility equipped to provide special care. Sometimes a high risk infant is transferred by ambulance or helicopter to a special facility after delivery.

IMPORTANT

Any of the following may be a sign that you are at risk for pre-term labor and delivery. Call your doctor immediately, and be prepared to go straight to the hospital if required.

****persistent or rhythmic low back pain that feels different from what you are used to in this pregnancy**
****menstrual-like cramps**
****intestinal cramps with or without diarrhea.**
****pelvic pressure or rhythmic tightening that feels different from what you are used to in this pregnancy**
****watery discharge or a gush of fluid from your vagina**
****vaginal bleeding**

WHEN THE BABY IS OVERDUE

How Long Is Too Long?

If your expected due date has come and gone, you're likely to be somewhat anxious, as well as certain you've been pregnant too long. When you feel as if the baby will never arrive, remember that the due date is only an estimate, and delivery two weeks earlier or later may be considered on schedule. And, there's always the possibility that an irregularity in your cycle might have caused a miscalculation. Chances are you're not really overdue and your baby will arrive when he or she is ready. Nevertheless, a few women do not go into labor at term as they should, and medical intervention may be required to prevent the baby from being seriously postmature.

What Can Be Done?

If you are more than two weeks past your expected due date, and you show no signs of labor, there are steps your doctor might take to make sure avoidable problems are prevented. There are several tests which might be used to assess fetal wellbeing. Which ones, if any, are used would depend on the particular circumstances of your case. Depending on the results of these tests, labor might be induced or your baby delivered by Caesarean section. Or, you might be reassured that everything is in order and you should wait a while longer. Feel free to ask any questions you might have, and share your concerns with your doctor.

You might want to go back and reread "When is the Baby Due?" on page 2. In FOR YOUR INFORMATION, pages 47-71, see the sections on AMNIOCENTESIS, ESTRIOL TESTS, INDUCED LABOR, NONSTRESS TESTS, OXYTOCIN CHALLENGE TEST, and ULTRASOUND.

SIGNS OF LABOR

Any or all of these three signs — contractions, rupture of membranes, bloody "show" can signal the beginning of labor.

CONTRACTIONS

During the last weeks of pregnancy, you may from time to time feel contractions of your uterus. These contractions, called Braxton-Hicks contractions, prepare the muscles for labor but do not result in the baby's birth. They do not become stronger with time, and generally can be relieved by a change in position.

The contractions of labor are different. When contractions come at regular intervals, increase in frequency, duration, and intensity as time progresses, and are not relieved if you lie down, you may be in labor. These contractions are characterized by a dull ache across the back which radiates around to the front. They may be accompanied by a sense of pressure in the pelvis.

RUPTURE OF MEMBRANES

The rupture of membranes, also called the breaking of the bag of waters, may be a sudden gush or a slow leak. The fluid is usually clear or slightly milky in appearance. It may be sticky, and it has little or no odor. Once the membranes rupture, you can not stop the flow the way you could control the flow of urine. There is no pain when the membranes rupture, although some women say they sense a tiny "pop." The membranes do not always rupture early in labor. It is possible for a baby to be born with the bag of waters still intact.

If your bag of waters breaks, and labor does not begin, be sure to tell your doctor. There is an increased chance of infection at this time.

"SHOW"

The mucous plug, which closes off the entrance to your uterus while you are pregnant, may be expelled just prior to or during labor. This is a small mucous mass, usually tinged with a little blood. It is often referred to as "show." It's appearance indicates that labor is likely to begin soon.

THE WAITING IS OVER

WHEN SHOULD WE CALL THE DOCTOR OR MIDWIFE?

If you suspect that any of the signs of labor are happening and would like to discuss them with your doctor or midwife, feel free to call. It's best if you can make the call yourself, rather than have someone else make it for you. This way you will be able to answer questions directly and explain exactly how you feel. High risk mothers should notify their prenatal caregivers promptly when labor begins.

IMPORTANT PHONE NUMBERS

Doctor/Midwife ______________________________

Hospital ______________________________

Taxi ______________________________

WHEN SHOULD WE LEAVE FOR THE HOSPITAL?

When you call, your doctor or midwife will discuss your condition with you on the phone, and perhaps see you in the office for a labor check. The time you should leave for the hospital will depend on how you are feeling, how your labor is progressing, and any particular circumstances of your case. Discuss with your doctor or midwife in advance what guidelines will be used for deciding when you should be admitted to the hospital. Be prepared to be flexible if unforseen circumstances signal a change in plans.

WHAT TO BRING

Don't make elaborate preparations for your hospital stay. It's likely to be short. For labor and delivery, you'll be wearing a hospital gown. A pair of cotton socks might be helpful in case you get chilly feet during labor. Bring something for your partner to eat, especially if you'll be in labor at a time when the cafeteria is closed. Leave expensive jewelry at home.

For your stay in maternity, you'll need clothing to keep you comfortable and covered as you wander between your room and the nursery. Bring something—slippers or moccasins—for your feet. If you're going to breastfeed, be sure that your gowns and robe open easily in the front. A lightweight robe with a front zipper is very handy. Don't forget your nursing bras—at least two. Bring your toothbrush, comb, and whatever makeup you'll want to use. If you're reading a good book, bring that along too. Don't make a big deal out of packing. Someone can bring you the things you've forgotten.

Delivery won't restore you instantly to your pre-pregnancy shape, so don't pack a garment that fits snugly for the trip home from the hospital.

THE HOSPITAL ADMISSIONS OFFICE

If your prenatal caregivers know that you are on the way, it's likely that the hospital will have been notified to expect you. You should find out ahead of time which entrance to use, what the admissions procedures are, and what financial arrangements are necessary. These are not matters you'll want to spend time figuring out when you are well along in labor, particularly if it's in the middle of the night.

Many hospitals have pre-admission procedures which enable you to complete much of the paperwork in advance. It's definitely better to take care of these matters before the need is urgent.

WHAT HAPPENS NEXT?

After being admitted to the hospital, you will go to the place where you are to spend your time in labor. In a hospital facility using traditional labor, delivery, and recovery rooms, you will be sent to the labor area. If you plan to labor and deliver in a private birthing room, you will go directly there.

Your nurse will give you a hospital gown to put on. She will ask you for a urine sample. If you have not had a recent bowel movement, an enema may be suggested. (See ENEMA, page 57.) If a prep has been ordered and you agree to this, it will be done at this time. (See PREP, page 61.) If you have any questions about these procedures, you should ask. if you choose not to undergo some of these routine admissions procedures, it's best to discuss your wishes with your doctor or midwife before you enter the hospital or labor.

In many birth settings it is possible for your partner to remain with you at all times, although staff in some hospitals prefer not to permit this. This is another point that you might wish to discuss with your birth attendant before the time comes. If you and your partner must be separated for any reason, be sure he knows where to find you as soon as you are settled.

The labor nurse will listen to your baby's heartbeat. Your temperature will be taken and your blood pressure will be checked. An internal examination will probably be done at this time to see how your labor is progressing. If your labor is going to be monitored electronically, the monitoring device will be set up. (See ELECTRONIC FETAL MONITORING, page 56.) If you are not monitored electronically, your baby's heartbeat will be checked frequently with a stethoscope. As your labor continues, you will be given an internal exam from time to time.

If you are to have your baby in the delivery room, you will be moved there a few mnutes before the baby is to be born. If you are in a birthing room, you will stay right where you are. For a detailed description of the stages of labor, see pages 84-89.

GUIDELINES FOR LABOR AND DELIVERY*

The following guidelines for labor and delivery are based on the reported experiences of many women. These descriptions will acquaint you with a typical labor and delivery and give you some idea of what might be in store. Do not, however, expect your labor to duplicate exactly what is described here. You may not experience all of the reactions listed and you may have some that are not mentioned.

The suggestions outlined here are very brief. They are not intended to replace classes for prepared childbirth or directions from your doctor. Reading this material should not make you feel that you must diagnose your own progress or that you have in some way failed if your labor does not fit the norm. No matter how well prepared you and your partner may be, you would do well to rely on the guidance of your birth attendants who will help you meet the personal demands of your particular situation as it evolves.

FIRST STAGE OF LABOR 0 to 2-3 cm. dilation

WHAT'S HAPPENING

The contractions are rhythmic and get stronger as time progresses. Women have described these contractions in a number of different ways, for example: as pelvic pressure, backache, like menstrual cramps, gas, tightening in the area of the pubic bone.

This stage of labor may also be accompanied by bloody show and/or rupture of the membranes. Some women feel chilly or experience nausea at this time.

For most women, this stage is the longest in comparison to the others. It may last several hours.

REACTIONS OF MOTHER

Because these signs indicate that labor is at last underway, most women feel excited and relieved, although these feelings are often accompanied by some measure of anxiety. Many women feel quite sociable at this stage and carry on conversation between contractions.

WHAT TO DO

- Indulge in activities to keep your mind off the contractions. Don't dwell on them. Try to think about other things.
- If it's nighttime or you're tired, it's fine to try to sleep.
- Read, watch television, or do something around the house to keep you busy as long as you feel able.
- If you think the contractions are 6-7 minutes apart or less, time them. Keep track of how often they occur and how long each one lasts.

HINTS FOR HELPING

- Encourage activities to keep her mind off the contractions.
- If she wants to rest, encourage her to do so.
- Take a walk with her.

*The material in this section was supplied by Barbara M. Perkins, RN

- Don't suggest timing the contractions until they are 6-7 minutes apart or less. If they are further apart than this, you shouldn't be in a hurry to focus attention on them.
- Make sure that things are packed and ready for the hospital trip, but don't rush off yet. Particularly with a first baby, this stage may take a long time.

FIRST STAGE OF LABOR 3-4 cm. dilation

WHAT'S HAPPENING

The contractions have become stronger and more regular. They are becoming increasingly uncomfortable.

REACTIONS OF MOTHER

As the contractions increase in intensity, many women don't feel like talking anymore. They become thoughtful and quiet. Although generally preoccupied with the labor and with self, most women need to know that someone is with them. Companionship rather than conversation is needed at this time. Talking during contractions is avoided. Although many women don't feel like walking around anymore, some still find it helpful.

WHAT TO DO

- Try to relax in a comfortable position (side or back) and change it every hour or so.
- Stay with normal breathing during contractions as long as possible. That way you'll feel that you still have some resources in reserve. Breathe slowly.
- Rest between contractions.
- Urinate, if you can, every 3-4 hours during labor.

HINTS FOR HELPING

- Help promote a relaxed, quiet environment. Avoid bright lights, unnecessary noise or commotion in the room.
- Provide continuous encouragement and reassurance.
- Don't invite the whole family. Too much company, no matter how well intentioned, will only get in the way.
- The doctor probably has given you guidelines for when to call. If this is the time, see that it's done. It's best if the person in labor talks to the doctor directly.

FIRST STAGE OF LABOR 5-8 cm. dilation

WHAT'S HAPPENING

Contractions are more frequent now. The peak of a contraction will be reached more quickly and it lasts longer. At this point, most laboring women are in contact with their doctor and in the hospital.

REACTIONS OF MOTHER

As labor reaches this stage, most women are very serious. Doubts about the ability to cope with the contractions yet to come are not unusual.

WHAT TO DO

- Begin using your controlled breathing techniques if you have not already done so. Stay with the deep chest breathing as long as you can.
- Some women may require medication to aid relaxation at this time.

HINTS FOR HELPING

- Offer words of encouragement. Things may be getting tougher to handle.
- Coach her on the controlled breathing through each contraction.
- Offer to supply pressure on her back to relieve backache.

FIRST STAGE OF LABOR 8- 10 cm. dilation (transition)

WHAT'S HAPPENING

Very pronounced contractions are coming on quickly, one after another. To many women these contractions feel continuous. There may be drowsiness between them. The abdominal wall is tense and many women feel unable to relax. Hiccups or belching, and a feeling of nausea and desire to vomit are not uncommon during this stage. Some women feel hot. Others feel cold. The legs may tremble and feelings of restlessness persist. Many women have beads of perspiration on the brow or upper lip.

REACTIONS OF MOTHER

Most women at this time are extremely sensitive and irritable. They may be short tempered and snap at people. Many women are surprised by the strength of the contractions at this stage. Their inability to relax frightens and frustrates them. This is a time that some women experience a feeling of panic and temporarily lose control. Expressions of discouragement and requests for help are frequent during this stage of labor.

WHAT TO DO

- Remember that this is the toughest part of labor for most women. It doesn't last very long even though at the time, it may seem eternal.
- Keep your eyes open during the contractions. Look at the focal point you selected, and concentrate.
- Think of one contraction at a time. Look forward to the rest, however brief, after it.
- Try shallow chest breathing for this stage.
- A cool damp cloth for the face and neck might help.
- If the mouth is dry, something wet — a damp cloth or ice chips — may help.
- Changes in position occasionally help during this transition.

HINTS FOR HELPING

- Provide constant reassurance that the feelings of getting out of control at this stage are normal reactions to the intensity of the contractions.
- Guide her through each contraction. As you talk her through it, be firm and encouraging. Direct her in her breathing.

- Remind her that this stage is short. It will end.
- Remind her to think of just one contraction at a time. Get through this one. Don't worry about the next.
- Remind her to rest between contractions.
- Offer something cool and wet (ice chips) for dry mouth.
- Wipe her face and neck with a cool washcloth.

FIRST STAGE OF LABOR
as transition nears its end

WHAT'S HAPPENING

As the transition stage nears its close, pain in the lower back will probably increase. It will be more difficult to continue the shallow chest breathing, and the urge to push may become strong.

REACTION OF THE MOTHER

At this time, many women feel a conflict between the need to continue chest breathing and the need to begin pushing. This confusion is quite common.

WHAT TO DO

- Try to listen carefully to instructions from your coach, even though it may be difficult at this time.
- Continue shallow chest breathing with blow until you are instructed to push or the urge can't be contained.
- Tell attending staff (doctor, nurse, or midwife) of urge to push.
- Try pressure on the lower back to relieve backache.

HINTS FOR HELPING

- Remind her not to push until it's time.
- Apply pressure on the lower back.
- Continue to direct controlled breathing.

SECOND STAGE OF LABOR
pushing and expulsion

WHAT'S HAPPENING

There may be a very brief period of deep sleep as this stage begins. The contractions may be further apart than they were during the transition stage of labor. They are expulsive in nature and require great effort on the part of the mother.

REACTION OF MOTHER

Many women feel an almost unbelievable sense of physical force or power at this stage. There is often surprise at the rapid change in feelings from transition to pushing. There is an irresistible urge to push, and pushing for most women brings with it relief and a sense of satisfaction. Unmedicated women tend to be very much more alert at this stage and experience a new spurt of energy. Many women act and look at this stage as if they were having a bowel movement.

WHAT TO DO

- Ease gradually into pushing. Follow the guidance of your medical team.
- Try to rest completely between contractions.
- Don't be afraid of your feelings or embarrassed by them. Feelings of power and pleasure at this time are normal. Enjoy them if you can.

HINTS FOR HELPING

- Reassure her that her feelings are normal and acceptable.
- Provide guidance through each contraction and remind her to rest between them.
- Some women are embarrassed by the similarity of this stage of labor to having a bowel movement. They may be afraid to push because they worry about making a mess. Remind her that these feelings are normal and that no harm will come from any mess that might be made.

SECOND STAGE OF LABOR
from appearance of baby's head to birth

WHAT'S HAPPENING

In a normal presentation, the baby's head is visible first. "Crowning" is when the head bulges the perineum and does not move back from sight between pushing contractions. An episiotomy (incision in the perineum to enlarge the birth opening) may be done at this time. The head is born first, then the shoulders. After the shoulders are delivered, the rest of the baby slides out easily.

REACTIONS OF MOTHER

Most women at this time are totally absorbed in the job at hand. They are indifferent to anything else going on. Many are impatient. There is a strong desire to push. Most women become more alert at this time and eager to see the baby. Some women are overpowered by the pressure and discomfort at this time and become fearful. Listening to the team will pull you through if this happens to you.

WHAT TO DO

- It's important to follow the instructions of the medical staff.
- Let the birth attendant guide you in the pushing efforts. Easing the baby's head and shoulders out may help avoid unnecessary tearing.

HINTS FOR HELPING

- If birth is to take place in the delivery room, the mother will be moved at the beginning of this stage of labor. It's easier if she is permitted to move onto the delivery table between contractions.
- Encourage cooperation with the medical staff. Pushing as directed can make things easier.

THIRD STAGE OF LABOR
delivery of the placenta

WHAT'S HAPPENING

The contractions may stop temporarily after the baby is born. When they resume, they are usually painless. There may be a trickle or a gush of blood. Expulsion of the placenta follows. A feeling of pressure, but little or no pain is experienced.

REACTIONS OF MOTHER

At this point, most women are proud of their achievement. Some feel a burst of energy and are eager to see the baby. Most women are exhausted. Many are extremely hungry and thirsty. There is no "right" way to feel. A wide range of reactions can be expected.

WHAT TO DO

- The medical staff will assist you as needed during this stage.
- The episiotomy, if any, will be repaired at this time.
- While repairs are done, many doctors will let the baby rest on the mother's abdomen.
- Many mothers choose to try to nurse the baby at this time.

Baby's Name ______________________________

Date and Time of Arrival ______________________________

Weight ______________ **Length** ______________ **Sex** ______________

Apgar Scale

Item Tested	*0*	*1 point*	*2 points*
Heart Rate	absent	slow (less than 100 beats per minute)	100 beats or more per minute
Breathing	absent	slow or irregular	regular
Muscle Tone	limp	some motion of extremities	active motion
Skin Color	blue	pink body, blue extremities	pink all over
Reflex Response	absent	grimace	cry

At birth, and again when he baby is five minutes old, his or her condition will be rated in five areas on a scale of 0 to 2. This rating, named for Dr. Virginia Apgar, the physician who developed it, is known as the Apgar Scale. A score of 7 or more indicates that the baby is in good condition. Most babies score 7 or higher by the five minute check. Immediate intervention is required for a baby who scores 4 or less. The Apgar rating is an indication of how well a baby has come through the stress of labor and delivery, and is not a predictor of long-term health.

BABY CARE (delivery room)

As soon as a baby is born, he or she must make the transition from being totally dependent on the mother, to functioning independently. Your birth attendants will assist the baby, as needed, to make this transition. If the baby is having trouble breathing, helping him or her to breathe is a top priority. Mucus will be suctioned from the baby's breathing passages if necessary.

Because a mother's body temperature—which is what the newborn has been used to—is significantly higher than the temperature of the room, the baby must be kept warm. For warmth, the baby may be placed on your abdomen and a blanket used to cover you both. This way the two of you can continue to be close to each other while the placenta is delivered and the episiotomy, if you had one, is repaired.

To complete the baby's adjustment to life outside the mother, the umbilical cord must be cut. Some doctors prefer to clamp and cut the cord immediately after the baby is delivered. Others will wait until the cord has stopped pulsating before cutting it, unless there is some specific medical indication for doing this sooner in a particular case.

If you plan to breastfeed your baby, you may wish to offer your baby the breast while still in the delivery room or birthing room. The baby's sucking stimulates the uterus to contract and helps it to return to its normal size more quickly. If you would like to nurse your baby immediately after delivery, discuss this in advance with your birth attendants. A few hospitals still discourage this, and you may have to make your wishes known in advance.

If you are following Leboyer's procedures for a gentle birth, your baby will receive a warm bath soon after delivery. Some couples choose to use the bath as one means to involve the baby's father actively in the child's care right from the start.

Before you and your baby leave the delivery room or birthing room, the nurse will make a record of your baby's footprints, along with one or more of your fingerprints. She will place identification bracelets on your baby—one on an ankle and one on a wrist. You will receive an identical bracelet for your own wrist. The purpose of these procedures is, of course, to make sure that your baby is not mixed up with anyone else's child.

ADDITIONAL MEDICAL PROCEDURES

In most states, babies are required by law to receive medication in their eyes to prevent infection. Antibiotic ointment is now used for this purpose in many places in preference to the more irritating silver nitrate drops. Many birth attendants are willing to delay administration of any medication until after the parents have had a chance to hold their baby and enjoy eye contact with the baby as part of the bonding process. You may discuss in advance what eye medication will be used for your baby and when it will be administered.

In most hospitals, babies receive an injection of Vitamin K to help the blood in clotting. Some hospitals routinely administer penicillin to all newborns to help prevent a baby from contracting an infection in the hospital nursery. The baby's blood might be tested for PKU disease, a rare form of mental retardation which can be prevented if detected and treated early. Many pediatricians routinely order the baby's blood to be tested for bilirubin level.

CIRCUMCISION

If your baby is a boy, one of the first decisions you will have to make is whether or not to have him circumcised. Because circumcision has been such a widespread practice in this country, many parents are under the impression that it is a necessity and they must agree to have it done. However, this is not so. There is no medical reason for routine circumcision. Regular bathing prevents the same problems that circumcision prevents.

The decision to have your child circumcised is a personal choice. It's generally best to delay this procedure for at least 24 hours after the baby is born. Jewish ritual circumcision is done on the eighth day.

BABY CARE (nursery)

In the hospital, your baby will be watched closely for a while to make sure that all systems are working well. Because some newborns have difficulty regulating their own body temperature, a heated bed may be used for a while until the baby's body temperature is normal. Don't be afraid to ask about the procedures that are being followed for your baby.

At most hospitals, new babies are brought to their mothers for feeding whenever the baby seems to be hungry. Mothers are encouraged to feed their babies at least every four hours, and to allow two hours to pass between feedings if possible. This is true for bottle fed as well as for breast fed babies.

If you are nursing your baby and prefer not to have bottles of glucose and water offered to your child in the nursery, you should discuss this in advance with your baby's pediatrician who will make the appropriate notation on the baby's chart. Follow the same procedure if you do not want your baby to be given a pacifier in the nursery.

BABY'S DOCTOR

A pediatrician will visit the hospital nursery daily, unless there is a special reason to see your baby more often. During your stay in the hospital, the doctor will visit you and speak with you about your baby. Feel free to ask questions and discuss any procedures you don't understand.

During your pregnancy, it is a good idea to start thinking about the need for a pediatrician, and whom you will choose. Your obstetrician or midwife may be helpful in recommending a pediatrician whose views on babycare would be consistent with your expectations. If the physician who delivers your baby is in family practice, he or she may continue to care for both of you after delivery.

Many women visit one or more pediatricians before the baby arrives to ask questions and find out about their policies. An informed choice is likely to be better for everyone involved.

Name of Doctor ______________________________

Address ______________________________

Telephone ______________________________

NAMING YOUR BABY

Soon after your baby is born, a hospital staff member will contact you for information for the baby's birth certificate. If you have not yet decided on a name, you may leave the space for the name blank. Depending on the state in which you live, you have from ten days to seven years to record the child's name. Once a name is recorded on the birth certificate, it may take a court order to change it.

While many parents choose to have their child use the father's last name, some do not. Especially when the woman has kept her own surname in marriage, the parents may choose to give the child a hyphenated combination of the mother's name and the father's name. Sometimes only the mother's name is used. The child of unmarried parents usually uses the mother's surname, but this is not required. A child's surname need not be that of either parent as long as no fraud is intended.

If you are planning to do something unusual with your child's name, check ahead of time to find out what special regulations, if any, there are in the state in which you live. If you prefer not to name your baby in a traditional way, don't be intimidated by those who insist you must. Make sure the official records reflect your wishes.

YOUR CARE AFTER DELIVERY

You will be watched very carefully after your baby is born, especially for the first few hours after delivery. Your blood pressure will be taken several times, and your fundus (uterus) will be checked frequently to see if it is remaining firm. Your vaginal flow (lochia) will be checked to make sure it is not excessive.

If you are hungry after delivery, as many women are, don't be afraid to ask for something, even if it's not mealtime.

HOSPITAL STAY

The length of your hospital stay will be determined by many factors: your condition and the condition of your baby, your personal preferences, and the practices generally followed by your physician, your baby's pediatrician, and the hospital in which you give birth. The trend today is toward shorter hospital stays in cases where delivery was routine for both mother and baby. Many women are now leaving the hospital a day or two after delivery, with some choosing to leave less than 24 hours after the baby is born. Early discharge from the hospital is less costly than a longer stay, and many parents find adjusting to their new baby easier in the familiar setting of home. Others, however, may welcome the opportunity to enjoy the change of pace they find in a hospital setting for a day or two longer.

If you have a Caesarean delivery, your stay in the hospital will be somewhat longer than it would have been with a routine vaginal delivery. The average stay after a Caesarean is five days, although you may be able to leave sooner.

Discuss hospital stay with your doctor or midwife before your due date. Find out what you will be permitted to do if all goes well. Remember, however, that medical reasons may develop to keep you in the hospital longer than you would like, regardless of what arrangements were made in advance.

If you choose to leave the hospital soon after delivery, a home visit by a health care provider may be suggested to help you be sure that everything is going smoothly.

Section Six

POSTPARTUM CARE

Activities / Afterbirth Pains / Bathing / Breast Care / Caesarean Postpartum / Constipation and Hemorrhoids / Episiotomy Aftercare / Exercise / Family Planning / Lochia / Lovemaking / Postpartum "Blues" / Rest / Weight Loss / Your Postpartum Checkup / Important Warning Signs

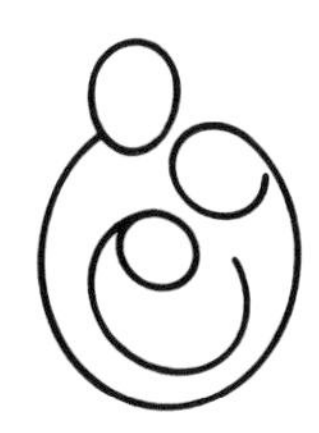

POSTPARTUM CARE

The following pages contain information on topics related to your own care after giving birth. Try to read these carefully before you leave the hospital so that you can discuss any questions you might have with your doctor. There is space below to note any special instructions for your particular situation.

Notes

ACTIVITIES

Common sense is an important ingredient in planning your activities during the first few weeks after your baby is born. If something seems to be a strain, skip it until you're better able. If you can get help with household chores, that's great. If you can't, leave everything but the absolute essentials. Forget about rearranging furniture or cleaning closets for a while.

Walking up or down stairs is fine when necessary, but you probably shouldn't carry anything heavier than your baby for the first week or two. If you have older children who want to be held, you can sit down and let them climb onto your lap rather than lifting them. Most women are quite able to drive a car and run short errands when they get home from the hospital. However, if you find yourself spending a lot of time doing such things you're probably not resting as much as you should be.

Rest (see page 98) is an essential part of your postpartum care. How much activity is comfortable and safe for you at first will depend on a number of things including how fit you were before and during your pregnancy, how difficult your delivery was, and any complications you might have had. While some women may feel able to ride a horse or play tennis a fortnight or so after delivery, most do not and should not. Before leaving the hospital, you should discuss with your doctor your plans for getting back to your normal activities. Find out which activities are fine for you right away, and which should wait until after your postpartum checkup.

AFTERBIRTH PAINS

As your uterus contracts after delivery, you may experience cramp-like feelings which are sometimes referred to as "afterpains" or "afterbirth pains." These contractions may cause some discomfort for a day or two. You are more likely to notice them if this is not your first baby, because your uterus will have to work harder to return to its prepregnancy condition.

During pregnancy, the uterus increases greatly in size. Right after delivery it will be about the size of a grapefruit. It will continue to get smaller each day until it has returned to its normal size. This process, called involution, takes about four to six weeks.

Breastfeeding helps to return the uterus to its normal size more quickly. If you are nursing your baby, you will be more likely to notice the afterbirth contractions in the first few days after delivery. If you find the afterpains bothersome, gentle massage or lying face down with a pillow under your abdomen may help.

BATHING

You will probably feel better if you keep your body as clean as possible after delivery. A daily shower is encouraged while you are in the hospital. Warm shallow baths will ease the soreness from hemorrhoids and episiotomy repair. Some doctors advise that patients avoid deep tub baths until three to four weeks after delivery to make sure that water doesn't enter unhealed body cavities. Others feel problems are so unlikely that such restrictions are not needed. If you prefer baths to showers, ask if there are any special reasons in your case that you should not take tub baths.

After delivery, the body uses its own natural cleansing process to rid you of waste blood, mucus, and other tissue. Your vaginal discharge at this time is a natural occurrence and douching is not necessary. Most physicians recommend that a woman not douche until after her postpartum checkup. Call your doctor if your vaginal discharge burns, irritates, or has a foul odor.

BREAST CARE

If you are breastfeeding your baby, you should use only warm water to keep your breasts clean. Avoid soap, which tends to dry out the nipples and cause them to crack. Be sure that your nursing bras are the right size and that they provide good support. If your breasts are sore, you may use lanolin on your nipples. Wipe off the excess with a tissue before your baby nurses.

If you are bottle feeding, you may receive medication to help dry up your milk supply. For a few days after delivery, your breasts may feel uncomfortable. Wrap ice cubes in a towel and apply to your breasts if they are engorged (full and swollen) or sore. An over-the-counter pain reliever may help you feel more comfortable. Ask your doctor for suggestions about what to take. Keep your breasts clean. You'll probably be more comfortable if you wear a bra that gives good support. If you are not nursing, don't express milk to relieve the fullness. This will stimulate your body to produce more.

If your breasts become red and painfully tender in spots, you should consult your doctor.

If you are nursing your baby and are having difficulty, a volunteer from La Leche League may be able to give you the support and encouragement you need to get by the early problems and nurse successfully.

CAESAREAN POSTPARTUM

If you deliver your baby by Caesarean, it will probably take you a bit longer to resume full activity than it might have otherwise. Remember, you have to recover from major surgery as well as cope with your newborn. A woman who delivers by Caesarean has a greater blood loss than one who delivers vaginally, and may need to be treated for anemia, which could prolong the convalescence somewhat. An average hospital stay after a Caesarean is five days, although your doctor may let you leave sooner or keep you longer, depending on your condition.

After a Caesarean delivery, you will be encouraged to get up and move around as soon as possible. Even if you don't feel like doing it, walking will improve your circulation, help prevent blood clots, and promote healing. Being in an upright position may help ease the intestinal gas pains that sometimes follow a Caesarean delivery.

The exercises to strengthen your abdominal muscles (see page 29) are very useful after a Caesarean. Ask your doctor when it is safe for you to begin these exercises. Begin slowly and work the time up very gradually. Stop if you feel pain or severe discomfort.

CONSTIPATION AND HEMORRHOIDS

Constipation is sometimes a problem for a new mother. Be sure your diet includes sufficient quantities of fluids and roughage. Try to relax. If you have soreness from an episiotomy or hemorrhoids, you may be afraid of trying to have a bowel movement. This fear can add to your problems. If you are having difficulty with constipation, be sure to report this. A laxative may be prescribed.

Many women have trouble with hemorrhoids after delivery. If this is a problem for you, be sure to tell your doctor or nurse. Appropriate medication can relieve the discomfort. Self-medication, however, may be unwise, particularly if you are breastfeeding.

EPISIOTOMY AFTERCARE

If you had an episiotomy, the stitches may feel sore or itchy at first. Here are some things that might help.

- Warm water may help. Try sitting in a warm shallow bath, or letting the water from the shower run over your perineum.
- A number of creams, sprays, or foam with local anesthetic are available. Apply one to your sanitary pad.
- Try cold Witch Hazel applied with a sterile gauze pad or cotton.
- You'll probably feel more comfortable sitting on something soft. If necessary, carry a small pillow with you and use it wherever you need to.
- Begin doing Kegel exercises immediately, even if this hurts at first. The exercises will help stimulate circulation in the perineal area and this will promote healing.

Perhaps most helpful is a positive attitude. If you fear moving about because you think it might hurt too much, it probably will. Don't dwell on the discomfort. Pretend it doesn't hurt when you do your exercises and walk around. Soon it won't. However if pain (rather than discomfort) persists, call your doctor. This may be a sign of complications and it should be checked out.

EXERCISE

Many of the exercises on pages 26-31 are useful after delivery to help you regain your muscle tone and energy. Many women, for example, can begin doing Kegel exercises and the exercise for separated abdominal muscles almost immediately. How quickly you will be able to begin an exercise program and resume your normal activities such as sports will, of course, depend on a number of factors — your fitness before delivery, any complications you might have had, your own motivation, and your body's ability to bounce back. You should discuss this with your doctor, and above all, use common sense. If it doesn't feel right, don't do it yet.

FAMILY PLANNING

The method of family planning you use should be a personal choice based on what is recommended as medically safe and effective for you, as well as what you find comfortable and consistent with your beliefs.

If you have just had a baby, here are some facts about family planning that you should keep in mind.

- It is possible to become pregnant again soon after your baby's birth, even if you have not yet had a menstrual period.
- Although many nursing women do not ovulate as long as they are breastfeeding, some do. Breastfeeding is not a reliable method of birth control.
- If your choice of family planning method is the diaphragm, it's likely that the one that worked for you in the past no longer fits. You can be measured for a new one at your postpartum checkup.
- If you are breastfeeding, you should not use oral contraceptives (birth control pills). They may decrease milk supply and the hormones from them can be passed to the baby in the milk.
- If you wish to use an IUD, it can be inserted when your uterus has returned to its normal size. Ask your doctor about this at your postpartum checkup.
- If you plan to get an IUD or a diaphragm at your postpartum checkup, but choose to resume sexual relations sooner, you may consider using condoms, foam, or jelly as directed for precaution during this interim time.

LOCHIA

Beginning right after delivery, a new mother experiences a vaginal flow called lochia. This is a normal process of cleansing. It continues until the place where the placenta was attached to the uterus has healed. For most women, the discharge lasts from a month to six weeks.

Lochia begins as a heavy flow similar in appearance to menstrual blood. At first, it is likely to contain clots, some of them quite large. The flow then turns brown, and then a yellowish white or colorless before stopping altogether.

Use sanitary pads, not tampons, and change them frequently. The pads provided in the hospital are individually wrapped in sterile packages, a useful precaution in the first days after delivery.

Keep yourself clean. Irrigate the perineum and outer vaginal area with warm water. (The squeeze bottle supplied by the hospital for this purpose makes a handy sprayer for plants when you no longer need it for you.) Wipe yourself gently from front to back, and only use each tissue once.

Especially at first, lochia may be a very heavy flow. How heavy is too heavy? If you soak through two pads in 30 minutes, or pass a clot larger than a lemon, report this to your doctor or a nurse. A flow which turns from brown back to bloody red should also be reported. This is often a sign that you have exerted yourself too much and temporarily interrupted the healing process.

LOVEMAKING

How soon after delivery can a couple have intercourse? There are no absolute answers to this question. It's probably best to wait three or four weeks while the vaginal wall muscles regain their strength and the episiotomy heals. You should ask your doctor whether there are any special circumstances in your case that might make waiting longer than this advisable. Some doctors advise that a woman wait until after her postpartum checkup to resume having intercourse.

At first, you may feel a bit uncomfortable because tissues are still tender. Talk to your partner about this. A slight change in position or a little extra gentleness may help. A lubricant such as K-Y Jelly may be helpful. Don't worry. Discomfort, if any, is a very temporary condition. It will pass.

If you are breastfeeding your baby, you might find that your breasts leak during intercourse. Don't be concerned. This slight flow of milk is a normal response to sexual excitement.

Remember that you could become pregnant again very soon after delivery unless you take specific precautions not to. Even if you have not had a menstrual period, you may have ovulated. Breastfeeding is not a means of contraception. It is possible to become pregnant while breastfeeding an infant.

It's best to discuss with your doctor what you will do about family planning before the need is urgent. This is a matter you would do well to consider before delivery, so you will be prepared when you need to be.

POSTPARTUM "BLUES"

You've probably heard people talk about the postpartum "blues," a condition that some women experience a short time after giving birth. If this feeling of unhappiness hits you, don't panic. No matter how delighted you are with your baby, it's possible to feel like crying for a few days. There are physiological reasons that this can happen. Feelings of depression often accompany the body's attempt to regain its fluid-salt balance after giving birth. For most women, this balance returns 4 to 7 days after delivery. For some it may take as long as ten days. If you feel overwhelmed by depression beyond this time, you should report it to your doctor.

REST

After you have had a baby, you may be extremely tired. Fatigue is a normal postpartum occurrence. Remember, your body has been under severe stress. You need time to recover.

Rest whenever you can. When your baby sleeps, you should too. Of course, this may be impossible if you have other young children. Common sense is the rule here. Don't take on unnecessary tasks until you are up to it. The house can do without cleaning for a while. You need not entertain or put your baby on display for acquaintances whose company drains your energy.

If you can afford household help, get some to do cleaning chores and laundry. The hired help should do the tasks that are drudgery. This will enable you to use what energy you have to take care of and enjoy your baby. When family and friends make demands that you are too tired to meet, remind them that the doctor has ordered you to rest. You'll never have a better excuse than you do now.

Be sure to take your iron supplement if one has been prescribed. Anemia is a frequent cause of fatigue in the days following delivery. If you are feeling extremely tired, and a reasonable amount of rest does not seem to help, give your doctor a call.

WEIGHT LOSS

If your weight gain has been within the recommended limit and from nutritious foods, you should be able to lose much or all of it by your postpartum checkup. Many women, particularly first time mothers, are surprised and disappointed to find that they don't come out of the delivery room slim and ready for their prepregnancy wardrobe.

During delivery you will shed the weight of your baby and approximately 1-1/2 pounds of placenta and between 1-1/2 and 2 pounds of amniotic fluid. The rest of the pregnancy weight gain will take a little longer, although you can probably get rid of much of the excess fluid within the first week or two. To lose the extra weight of your enlarged uterus and other tissue will take at least another month.

Right after your baby is born is not the time to go on a crash diet, no matter how motivated you may be to strive for thinness. Your body needs nutritious food to regain its strength and give you enough energy to care for your baby. Stay away from food fads and diet pills. You need a balanced diet. The suggestions on prenatal nutrition (pages 31 to 46) still hold. Foods high in protein will help you feel better and avoid putting on extra pounds.

If you were taking prenatal vitamins and an iron supplement during your pregnancy, you should continue this postpartum unless your doctor directs you otherwise. If you are breastfeeding, you will probably require up to 1000 additional calories of nutritious fluids and foods daily.

If you are maintaining a well-planned program of nutritious meals and adequate exercise, and your weight loss is still slower than you would like, talk to your doctor about it.

YOUR POSTPARTUM CHECKUP

Your first postpartum checkup is a very important one. The exact timing of this checkup will vary with your doctor's policies and your particular needs. It is likely to be four to six weeks after your baby is born. You may be seen sooner after a Caesarean delivery. At the postpartum checkup you will be examined to make sure that your uterus has returned to its normal size and position and that your episiotomy (if you had one) has healed. A pap smear and a breast examination may also be done at this visit. This is the time to ask your doctor any questions you still have about diet, vitamins, exercise, family planning, or other matters related to your personal health care and childbearing.

Although your doctor's office expects you for a postpartum checkup, it's still up to you to make the appointment. Call the office to reserve a time as soon as you can after leaving the hospital. Use the space on the next page to note the date and time for your appointment and any questions you have for the doctor.

POSTPARTUM CHECKUP

Date ______________________________ Time __________________________

QUESTIONS FOR THE DOCTOR

IMPORTANT

Don't wait until your postpartum checkup to ask for help if you experience any of the following:

**trouble with your bowels, your breasts, or your bottom
**bleeding heavier than a period
**chills or fever
**pain
**persistent headaches
**dizzy spells
**severe depression

Call your doctor right away if you are bothered by any of these problems.

INDEX

Additional copies of **While Waiting** or any of the St. Martin's Press perinatal care books recommended on pages 72–75 may be purchased from most booksellers or by mail on the order form below. Substantial discounts on orders of 10 or more books are available to physicians, clinics, midwives, childbirth educators, and individuals. For information, call: St. Martin's Press, Special Sales Dept. Toll Free (800) 221-7945. In New York (212) 674-5151.

Order Form:	Copies	Price
While Waiting: A Prenatal Guidebook ($5.95) (867735)	______	______
Mientras Espera ($4.95) (Spanish-language edition of *While Waiting*) (01791X)	______	______
Welcome Baby: A Guide to the First Six Weeks ($5.95) (861214)	______	______
Talk & Toddle: A Commonsense Guide for the First Three Years ($7.95) (784309)	______	______
Breastfeeding and the Working Mother ($9.95) (095279)	______	______
Babysense ($9.95) (064586)	______	______
Giving Birth ($12.95) (01032X)	______	______
Having a Baby ($10.95) (364369)	______	______
The Parents' Guide to Raising Twins ($15.95) (596618)	______	______
Time Out for Motherhood ($8.95) (0-87477-449-7)	______	______
Postage and handling: $1.50 for first book and 75¢ for each additional book.		______
Amount enclosed:		________

Name ____

Address ____

City/State/Zip ____

Send this form with payment to St. Martin's Press / Special Sales Dept. / 175 Fifth Ave. / New York, NY 10010. Please allow three weeks for delivery.